WHAT PROFESSIONALS ARE SAYING
ABOUT THIS BOOK

"This wonderful book of deep wisdom is both inspirational and informative. It is a guide to bountiful, joyous, living in a troubled world."

"Hopefully, it will encourage readers to take the Kalos Seminars, which puts healing precepts into dynamic practice. I have found the information and skills learned there to be of great value in my profession."

Claudia MacDorman, C.A.
Licensed Acupuncturist, Encinitas, CA

"As a chiropractor and a holistic health care provider I have found the information in this book invaluable in the management of illnesses and structural problems that just won't respond to treatment. I recommend this book to anyone desiring to release themselves from chronic nagging health problems and to professionals including ministers, psychologists, medical doctors, and alternative health care providers who really want to help their patients. Emotions play such a major role in the drama of life and truly inhibit the healing processes; Valerie has found an **easy, gentle, and effective** way to penetrate the subconscious to speed up emotional release."

Cynthia Leeder, D.C., M.S.
Applied Kinesiologist,
Masters in Bio-Nutrition, Oceanside, CA

"Reading this reminds me of why I love Valerie. Your wisdom comes through with the simplicity of truth. Understandable and yet thought provoking. This will help a lot of people get their "healings."

"I thank you for making this work available to all who reach out for it, for leading me into the healing of cancer (It's now five years after a stage III cancer and no invasive procedures), healing of finances, relationships and Spiritual discontent."

"This book is like listening to Valerie teach, share and prod us into stretching our "comfort zones" into increased health and well-being."

The Rev. Sara Schmidlin, Ph.D.
Psychologist - Private Practice, Atlanta, GA

"This book differs from the many others on healing and is long overdue. The techniques have proven to be powerfully effective. They enable the reader to strike at the heart of physical, emotional and spiritual health and eliminate the blocks. I love the process and the work."

Dorothy Dumbra, R.N.,
Applied Kinesiologist, Citrus Heights, CA

"Valerie is introspectively guiding us 'with love' toward health. The disease or the symptom becomes a message of imbalance between our thoughts, our values, our emotions, and our behavior. The body reflects these contradictions in sickness. This book will interest everyone who is open to be in the forefront of transformation including health professionals."

Elisabeth Reichel, M.D.,
Homeopath, P.N.C., Montreal, Canada

A New Day in Healing!

Principles & Practices for Creating Health

By

Valerie Seeman Moreton, N.D.

KALOS^{SM} *TRANSFORMATIONAL HEALING*
BOOK ONE

KALOS PUBLISHING,
SAN DIEGO, CALIFORNIA

A NEW DAY IN HEALING!
Principles and Practices for Creating Health
By Valerie Seeman Moreton, N. D.

Kalos™ Transformational Healing, Book One

Published by:

Kalos™ Publishing
P.O. BOX 270817
San Diego, CA. 92188-2817

❋ This book printed in the USA on recycled, archival-quality paper

Typesetting/Cover Layout by Ben Cravy, BusinessType, Escondido, CA
Cover Photo by Douglas Moreton

Publisher's Cataloging in Publication
Moreton, Valerie Seeman. 1938-
A new day in healing!: principles and practices for creating
health / by Valerie Seaman Moreton. 1st ed.
p. cm. -- (Kalos transformational healing; bk. 1)
includes index
ISBN 1-882590-01-5: $12:00 Softcover

1. Naturopathy. 2. Mental Healing 3. Spiritual Healing I.
Title, II, Series

RZ440.M67 1992615.5'35
   QBI92-20062

Library of Congress Card Number 92-075049

See last page for ordering information

THIS BOOK IS DEDICATED TO

MY TEN PRECIOUS CHILDREN:

Don
Susanne
Wendy
Sharee
Cindy
Teri
Laurie
Matthew
Mark
Jaycie

Who motivated me to understand the laws of health and gave up valuable time together for the benefit of many.

IN APPRECIATION

TO THOSE WHO HELPED GET THIS BOOK TO YOU

A special big thanks to my husband, Douglas Moreton for his massive efforts to publish these works and promote health, happiness and harmony in our world.

Another special thank you to my partner and friend, Madeleine Houle, for her great support and motivation.

More thanks and appreciation to the many who contributed to the editing and final copy:

Peggy Allen, Paula Bergen, Gloria Latham, Joanne Magram, Lena McInerney, Teri Mister, Jane Nelson, Sandra Prior, June Schnell (my mother-in-law), Bill Silver, Max Skousen, Steve Stevens, and Jo Ellen Tropper.

A NEW DAY IN HEALING

TABLE OF CONTENTS

**KALOS TRANSFORMATIONAL HEALING
BOOK ONE**

DISCLAIMER

This book is sold with the understanding that the publisher and author are not engaged in rendering professional services or medical advice. This book does not take the place of the services of a competent health professional.

This book is not a treatment of any physical, mental or emotional illness. It is not a substitute for ongoing therapy (medical or psychological). It is not about giving advice on how to solve the problems of life. It is not about taking sides or establishing blame. It is not about deciding what is right or wrong. It is not a magic pill that guarantees the non-disturbed state. The theories and principles described in *A New Day in Healing* can assist YOU in creating profound differences in your life. It is your responsibility to make sure you utilize these concepts and methods with discretion.

Every effort has been made to make this manual a complete and accurate introduction to the possibility of being healed. However, there may be mistakes both typographical and in content. Therefore, this text should be used only as a general guide and not as the ultimate source of information on transformational healing. Furthermore, this manual contains information only up to the printing date.

The purpose of this manual is to educate and inform. The author and Kalos Publishing shall have neither liability nor responsibility to any person or entity with respect to any loss or damage caused, or alleged to be caused, directly or indirectly by the information contained in this book.

If you do not wish to be bound by the above, you may return this book to the publisher for a full refund.

PREFACE

"God loves you and wants you to be well!" This message is to all people who want healing in any area of their life. Whether you have a physical, mental, emotional or spiritual problem, you will need to get to the source of the problem to have complete victory and permanent health. Otherwise, old problems may return in the same or similar way.

God really does love you and wants you well. Complete healing IS a wholistic event and must include spiritual insights and awareness beyond the physical domain. There are laws that govern all aspects of our being; physical laws, mental laws and moral laws. To keep healing restricted to the physical laws limits the healing. Permanent health is freedom. Potential health is within us all.

Every person has a gift to bring to others. Every soul is unique and special. The gift I bring is for healing. I prayed for years to understand the laws of health and wholeness. This book is a composite of my experiences in pursuit of that understanding. My gift is to share wholistic healing in as pure a form as I can. Wholistic means whole. It begins with a "W" because it includes physical health as well as going beyond to the mental and spiritual realms.

It is my wish that the terminology used will be understood by all. I have used many universal terms, so that more people are reached and served. I encourage you to translate the terminology into your own. Make it as easy as possible to understand.

This book is part of a work that compiles twenty-five years of research and exploration to understand the laws of health and HEAL THE CAUSE of physical and emotional disease. The methods are taught by Kalos Seminars

International to lay people and professionals (in English and French), who want a NEW DAY in healing. Though comprehensive in nature, these methods are noted for being the fastest way to heal.

This book is meant to alert people to the possibilities of healing themselves, especially where there is no known cause. You can learn to dynamically take charge of your health; you can then assist others to do the same. The technology is here to succeed.

The Kalos theories and techniques come from many methodologies, philosophies and personal explorations in healing that I have found effective. Kalos is a comprehensive approach to healing, yet it is in a form that the lay person can put to use immediately. Within the pages of this book are insights for you to begin the healing process right now.

While this book focuses on the mental, emotional and spiritual aspects of healing, Book Two introduces the Kalos Process itself. In addition, Book Three, The Manual, describes the step by step methods using multiple modalities, including reading the body at a cellular level through Muscle Response Testing. We invite you to investigate all the books in the series.

You don't have to buy any equipment or have a college degree. Your body holds all the answers and all the data needed to understand and resolve your problems. Your mind is like a highly sophisticated, bio-electrical computer. It is complete with accessible records and analytical assessments. In tracing a problem to its cause you can uncover when and why it began. Every bit of information from every age of your life is stored inside.

Your mind can sift through all this data to find the related information on every aspect of a problem you are seeking to understand. You can determine what emotions are locked in your body and what personal or family patterns are involved.

In every case of chronic illness I find unresolved emotions perpetuating the problem. Emotions that get trapped in your body can cause physical pain and long lasting illnesses. They can attach themselves to fungal, bacterial and viral infections of all types, making recovery difficult, if not impossible. You can learn to determine what those emotions are and how to release them from your body. I find that how one deals with stress is the biggest factor influencing your health. Healing your emotions is the major part of this book. Even though you may not have a specific problem, there is always an area of your life to improve upon. It can be a fascinating journey!

It is my hope that you will support your wellness by answering the questions and filling in the requests on the "Participant's Pages" as you move through the chapters. You transform your life as you get honest and clarify the truth. Be as specific as possible so your mind can best support you. Like a seed planted in fertile ground, allow your faith to explore and abound.

The Holy Spirit lit a spark in me that turned into a burning desire and guided my investigation into wholeness. May your prayer join with mine:

"God, help me to understand the laws of health
and be an instrument for HEALING."

I deeply appreciate the many teachers, patients and students who helped make this a working reality. I am grateful to God for planting the seed of research in my heart. I thank you for seeking to understand - that you can create health, happiness and harmony in our world.

Author

Chapter One

Stop!
You Don't Have to Suffer

Millions of people are suffering needlessly from pain, illness, low energy, and emotional difficulties. Many others are feeling defeated in some area of their lives.

There is an Answer

My heart wants to cry out STOP! There is an answer to your problems. You don't have to suffer! You can do something to regenerate your body, raise your energy, end your pain, defuse your emotions and take charge of your life.

Not long ago on a return flight from the East Coast, I read a lengthy article on arthritis. There were pictures of people in wheel chairs learning to cope with their defeated way of life. This brought tears to my eyes as I felt those hearts ache. I was a bit embarrassed as a lump came in my throat. I wanted to cry out to those people STOP! You don't realize that you can be healed! It has been difficult for me to sit back and watch the defeatism going on where victory could prevail.

There are No Incurable Diseases

I have seen people leave their wheel chairs and their crutches behind. I have seen every kind of disease healed. God has given me a reverence for the human body and a confidence in the body's ability to heal and repair itself. Problems show up because of broken natural laws. The body then has to make alterations to preserve our lives. If the body places something in itself, such as a tumor, it can remove it. *What the body creates, it can take away.* I believe the answers were created before the problems became possible. I believe in that kind of a loving Creator who works with natural laws as well as spiritual laws. I could not love and adore a God who was less than that. You can master your health, as you align yourself to those natural and spiritual laws. It is your birthright. It is God's promise to you.

Disease is a Result of Breaking Natural Laws

You wouldn't think of jumping off a ten story building unless you wanted to commit suicide. You know that the law of gravity would pull you downward to death. The same is true for the laws of health. You cannot break them without suffering the consequences. Disease, fatigue and premature death are the result.

This book is the first of a series to assist you to align your life with life's natural laws. You can learn how your body and mind works. You can open up and explore your body's ability to repair itself. Your confidence in the healing process will grow as you align yourself to natural laws. You first may need to align your mind to "thinking" and "feeling" that you want to be healed and that it is possible to be healed. Knowing for sure that God wants you well will aid the process. This volume of the "Be Healed" series relates to how your mind works and affects your health. Without aligning your mind on a conscious and subconscious level, you may reprogram old problems back again. Your mind controls your body mostly from a subconscious level. Permanent healing, not band-aid therapy is our aim.

Pray for Clarity

I request that you pray while reading this book; that God will manifest to you what is His perfect Will for your life. I am not referring to a detached, unreachable God, but to the very Life and Essence within you. "There is . . . one God and Father of all who is above all, and through all, and in you all." (Ephesians 4:6) I want to challenge you to get really honest about whether or not you believe God wants you well or sick. Also, do YOU really want to get well?

Are you deceived into believing you must have ailments or diseases to transcend to the next life? Can you choose to live healthily and leave this world naturally? Less than two percent of the people in America die of a natural cause, whereas more than ninety percent die of natural causes in some less civilized places in South America.

I remember the first time I saw someone transcend naturally (without a physical reason). Mr. Condie was a sweet old man in his late nineties. He got up one day in front of the church and told everyone it was time to say good-bye. He was in fine health, but felt he wanted to cross over to where his wife and other loved ones were. He said he was leaving to visit his family out of state to say good bye to them and tell them he loved them before he departed. Three months later I got word he died in his sleep very peacefully. As you can see, you don't need a disease to die, so surely you don't need one to live!

The Body Does Not Make Mistakes – Only Compensations

Presumptions have been made in the past that the body makes mistakes and works against us. We were told to "compensate for the body's mistakes" through medicines and surgery and that if we were fortunate, the symptoms would be relieved, but not the cause. In this process, many people have had reactions to certain drugs, which in turn have caused other problems. I am grateful for many life saving medicines, as well as the physician's scalpel, but too many times they are used because no other method of healing is known. Within these pages we offer a fresh look at healing. The new technology employs a different premise: the body does not make mistakes. In fact, it is always working FOR us. The body is marvelously made to repair itself, if given the chance. I believe everyone is blessed by God already with a body that can automatically heal itself if the cause of the disease is identified and stopped. Healing is the natural state for everyone.

Science is now conscious of how the body adjusts for our welfare.

Your body is continually doing everything to preserve your life. It makes alterations to keep the Life blood flowing and the vital organs functioning with as much ease as possible. When one breaks natural laws the body struggles to keep you well and in balance.

8

Forcing the body through the use of drugs only masks symptoms, sometimes to the extent that an underlying ailment is overlooked. Pain relievers intercept messages to the brain that a part of the body needs help. However, you don't have to wonder or worry about what caused your problem any more because *one can now ASK what caused the body to get sick and what it needs to get well.* You can be the major factor in your healing process. If you are working with doctors, let them know you want to take an active role in your healing process and get to the source of the problem. If possible, work with a health professional who knows how to trace your problem to its cause. By using Applied Kinesiology you can uncover hidden cellular information and find the underlying cause of any problem. You can locate a kinesiologist in your area to assist you, or come to a Kalos Training Seminar. You will want some hands-on help to make sure the testing is accurate. You really can take greater charge of your health, more than you ever dreamed possible. Learning how your mind works will be a big step in this process.

You can be in Charge of Your Healing Process

You can uncover the root cause of your problem and resolve it. I am not suggesting that you no longer consult a physician. What I am saying is that you can participate in getting well and staying well. You have a body that repairs itself automatically, if given the chance. Do not stop any medication without consulting your physician. Most medications must be eliminated very slowly, so you do not have an adverse reaction. Speak freely to your health advisor to gain an understanding of why you are taking certain drugs. Your doctors will tell you that drugs don't heal. Doctors know

9

that drugs only attempt to compensate for what they feel the body cannot do on its own.

There is an adage that has been around the medical schools a long time: "The doctor entertains the patient, while nature either kills or cures." Though this has been a long-standing joke, there is much truth to it. Healing is an "inside job," inside you! Spirit heals, the mind directs, and the body restores.

The chapters to follow will be for your exploration and healing. May the seed of faith be planted for your success.

Highlights

* There is an answer to your problem. You don't have to suffer.

* There are no incurable diseases. God wants you well. The answers were here before the problem.

* Disease is a result of breaking natural laws. Healing is a result of aligning yourself to the laws of health.

* Pray while reading this text and seek God's Will for yourself. Become clear and know that God wants you well.

* Health is your natural state. The body is programmed to heal itself. It doesn't make mistakes as previously thought; instead it adjusts for our welfare.

* Your body can heal naturally by identifying and resolving the cause. The breaking of natural physical laws and moral laws are the basis of all disease.

* Eliminating symptoms without taking care of the cause can be dangerous and lead to other problems. Symptoms are adjustments the body makes to keep your life going. Listen to them.

* You can be in charge of your healing process by uncovering the cause of your disease and resolving it.

* Use common sense and wisdom in your healing process. Do not stop any medication without consulting your physician.

* You can take an active role in your healing process. Healing is an "inside job." Spirit heals, mind directs, and the body restores.

Participant's Page

It is my wish that you will allow inner guidance to show you the way, as you participate in your own "book of life." Trust that you can make a difference in your life. Are you ready to take the responsibility for your life? Responsibility means "the ability to respond." Only you can do that. There are no magic pills outside of you. God in you is powerful and God made you able to heal yourself.

1. WRITE DOWN A SPECIFIC PROBLEM THAT YOU WOULD LIKE ANSWERED BY THE TIME YOU FINISH THIS BOOK. BE CLEAR AND SPECIFIC. LIST MORE THAN ONE IF YOU WISH.

2. ASK YOURSELF: "DO I REALLY WANT TO GET RID OF THIS PROBLEM?" HONESTY IS IMPORTANT. IS THERE ANY HIDDEN AGENDA LIKE: "IF I GET RID OF THIS PROBLEM, I'LL HAVE TO GO BACK TO A JOB I HATE" OR "OTHERS WILL EXPECT TOO MUCH OF ME." LOOK FOR WAYS YOUR LIFE WOULD CHANGE IF YOU NO LONGER HAD THE PROBLEM. DOES ANY FEAR SHOW UP?

3. LIST WAYS YOU HAVE BEEN BLESSED BY HAV-ING THIS PROBLEM. LOOK AT WAYS YOU HAVE COMPENSATED FOR IT. WHAT HAVE YOU LEARNED? HAVE YOU LEARNED ENOUGH? ARE YOU READY TO MOVE ON TO OTHER CHALLENG-ES?

4. WRITE DOWN WHY YOU BELIEVE YOU HAVE THIS PROBLEM. THEN CHECK AT THE END OF THE BOOK TO SEE IF YOU STILL FEEL THE SAME WAY.

5. PRAY DAILY FOR GUIDANCE IN YOUR HEALING PROCESS. ALIGN YOURSELF TO SPIRITUAL LAWS OF CONNECTEDNESS AND RESULTS.

Chapter Two

You Can Get to the Source of Your Problem

The principles and laws of health lie hidden beneath the surface. The challenge is setting aside all preconceived ideas of what caused your problem and look at new possibilities that go beyond the physical level into mental programming and beyond.

"The world we have made as a result of the
level of thinking we have done thus far,
creates problems we cannot solve at the same
level at which we created them."
                                        –Albert Einstein

Until we are willing to open our hearts and minds and look beyond the thinking of the past, we will not make a significant difference in our own health or the health on our planet. . . Everything in and around us points to the problems that lie well hidden beyond the physical realm. Rampant diseases, viruses of all types and many environmentally related problems are plaguing our day. Wellness

15

will require us to go beyond the limitations of the past, beyond the body, and even beyond the mind, to the source and to *understand those laws that are being broken.*

We need to uncover what we have called "cause" in the past and ask the next question: "And what caused that?" The Kalos Process helps you find and heal the root cause of physical and emotional problems.

There was a large, strong looking man who came to me with debilitating pain in his back. He had been in an automobile accident over three years earlier. At first glance I thought the cause was obviously his serious injury. He could hardly get up on the treatment table. "The pain has never gone away," he said, "only let up once in a while." He had tried pain relievers to little avail. Physical therapy and Chiropractic methods only relieved him a minimal amount. I expected to do some nerve and muscle work for relief, but much to my surprise, I never did any structural work on him at all. In testing what the body wanted as a priority for his healing, "Emotional release" came up first; so we did a Kalos Process.

In the Process he went back to the time of the accident and saw the truth anew of what and why it happened. Resentments and anger toward the other driver had brought up old resentments toward his father. The new resentments from the accident clustered together with old resentments from the past and settled in his lower back. He became misaligned to mental and spiritual laws through his judgment and resentment. Then he blamed his own problems on others. Would you believe a misalignment to natural law could bring a misalignment of his spine? What followed looked like a miracle.

After seeing what he had done, he took responsibility for his part of the accident and stopped blaming the other driver. He also took responsibility for how he distanced himself from his own father. His anger and resentment disappeared as he saw the truth of the matter and recognized he was not a victim unloved by God. It was beautiful to watch him connect with his father and get off the table without pain!

This level of healing made a difference in his happiness as well as his health. Today he enjoys a healed relationship with his father, as well as a strong back. Notice the spiritual law that was broken: "honor your father and mother, that your days may be long upon the earth."

Who would ever believe that not healing from an automobile accident could have anything to do with an unresolved resentment from youth. I never did any physical work on him and he left pain free. Furthermore, the pain never came back! This verified again that if we get to the underlying cause, the problem goes away.

Chronic Problems are Emotional Problems

In case after case I find that when a problem does not correct itself within a reasonable amount of time, it is because there are emotions trapped within the cells of the body causing inflammation and stress. It only takes a couple of weeks for the body to heal from most major surgeries, yet many suffer for months or years from the same ailment. I have never seen a chronic case of anything that didn't have some emotional block or pattern attached to it. Those emotional blocks can mask an even greater block beyond it - a broken spiritual law.

Your Body is a Barometer – Symptoms Are "Wake-Up" Calls

You have a body, but you are not your body. You have a mind, but you are not your mind. You are far more than these. You are spirit, created in the image of God. You are infused in a body/mind through which to express yourself through. The body shows you symptoms of problems, acting as a barometer to reveal your inner state. The cause of problems is rarely at a physical level.

The reason we have so many ailments and "incurable" diseases today is because the CAUSES are not resolved. The focus in healing has been on a physical or symptomatic level, instead of getting to the source. We wouldn't think of cleaning water off the floor UNLESS WE STOPPED THE LEAK. We would first turn off the water and fix the pipe. Treating symptoms and not the cause is similar to this.
Much of your fatigue and ill health is a "wake-up" call that you are breaking some natural or spiritual law. If you drive your car into a wall, you are going to get hurt. If you drive your emotions into the basement of your mind, you also will get hurt. Held hurts can surface to meet you in another place. Unforgiveness keeps you from an intimate relationship with God. When resentment and anger alienate you from your spiritual source, there is a tendency to feel unworthy of healing or happiness. This defeated attitude can interfere with your motivation in life and in your commitment to living your spiritual Purpose – the very reason for your existence! This fundamental component of health and well-being – your Purpose for living – is discussed more in later chapters.

Furthermore, since natural laws of cause and effect function on a spiritual plane, your lack of vitality may have to do with not living your spiritual Purpose. Clarify your Purpose and align your thinking to support it. You will recognize your Purpose by the joy and enthusiasm it brings. There is a fascinating journey awaiting filled with joy and vitality!

I speak of breaking natural and spiritual laws, but the truth is you can't. You can only break yourself against them. A law is something that doesn't change, it just is. You may try to change those natural laws. You may even convince yourself they do not exist, but the consequences are the same – you can only break yourself against them. Fatigue and illness are the result.

Illness May be Your Body Shouting at You!

That pain in your left shoulder is actually trying to tell you that something is out of balance in some area of your life. It may even be an unresolved issue from the past that is now able and ready to be healed. It is time to explore beyond the limitations of the past and be open to resolving problems at a causal level. Even accidents have a cause.

Worry has become one of the earth's major emotional plagues in our day. It comes out of fear, and from not trusting that we are loved and cared for. Worry gets trapped in the pancreas, the very organ that helps us maintain a normal blood sugar. Diabetes is the fastest growing disease in our nation. Worry isn't worth it.

I remember a charming elderly man who loved to compose music. His joy was to sit at his piano and play for hours. When I met him, he had not played this way for more than seven years. He could sit on the piano bench only a few minutes at a time because of nagging pain between his shoulder blades. He worried about losing this joy-filled ability in his now retired years. His wife told me that he had always been a big worrier.

In respect to the wife's request I provided a few minutes of therapeutic massage and the pain disappeared. He thought that a miracle had happened. Fixing the pain in his back was only treating the symptoms though. This did not stop the worry. This same man later created cancer in his chest out of worrying about a discomfort felt there, which actually was a hiatal hernia. When examined, he would not believe the doctors. He kept insisting that he had cancer there. Several years later he got the cancer right where he thought it to be.

There is a cause behind everything – every problem in your life.

Now you can learn to identify it:
   what is going on;
   who is involved;
   when it began to be a problem and exactly
   what the body/mind needs to resolve it.

Even more than problem solving, you can learn your "bottom line" programming that keeps problems from coming back. You can identify your mental "con game" that keeps getting you into trouble. You then can change how you think and transform your life by "the renewing of your mind." In fact, this is part of the blueprint to achieve a wonderful joy-filled life.

Highlights

* There are new ways to understand the cause of your problems. You can go beyond the surface to where the belief began.

* Chronic problems involve unresolved emotions that got trapped in your body. They can cause tension and pain.

* You can identify hidden resentments through the Kalos Process. When the mind sees the truth, it is set free.

* Your body speaks to you through pain and discomfort (Symptoms). I call them "wake-up" calls. The body wakes you up to look at whether you are breaking a natural or spiritual law.

* Spiritual laws of cause and effect may be a factor in your health. Living your spiritual purpose enhances your vitality.

* You cannot break natural laws; you can only break yourself against them.

* Your mind controls your body, as it does most areas of your life. Mental programming is at the core of most of your problems. You can change this by changing the way you THINK. You can transform your life by the renewing of your mind.

* There is a cause behind every problem in your life. You can learn what to do about it.

Participant's Page

1. LIST YOUR PHYSICAL AND/OR EMOTIONAL COMPLAINTS.

2. WRITE A PARAGRAPH ABOUT YOUR COMMIT-MENT TO RESOLVE YOUR PROBLEM. ARE YOU WILLING TO CHANGE YOUR UNHEALTHY HABITS AND SUPPORT YOUR WELL-BEING? (Example: "I know I need to stop smoking, drinking, eating sugar, complaining," etc.) Pick one at a time and ask your family to support you.

3. OWN YOUR PROBLEMS; DON'T BLAME ANYONE OR ANYTHING ELSE. JUST FOR NOW, PRETEND YOU WANTED THOSE COMPLAINTS FOR SOME BENEFIT IN YOUR LIFE. (Example: "I smoke because it makes me feel in control. I don't like others telling me what to do.")

4. CHOOSE TO LOVE YOURSELF THE WAY YOU ARE. USE UNDERSTANDING AND COMPASSION. FORGIVE YOURSELF, IF NEED BE, TO MAKE PEACE. (Example: "I appreciate wanting to be in control of my life. When I make decisions that support my well-being, I am in control of my life. I forgive myself for abusing my body and commit to taking care of it.")

5. IF APPROPRIATE, CONFESS ANY "WRONG-DOING" AND ASK FORGIVENESS. (Example: "I am sorry for my rebelliousness, seeking to control others, needing my own way," etc.)

6. MAKE RIGHT ANY WRONG-DOING AND SEEK TO UNDERSTAND WHY YOU ACTED THAT WAY. When you get to your core subconscious programming, you will deeply understand the cause of your behavior. Compassion will then replace self-guilt.

7. FOR THE NEXT FIVE DAYS, NOTICE WHAT PERCENTAGE OF THE TIME YOU ARE FEELING HAPPY AND SATISFIED WITH YOUR LIFE. Notice how much better you feel about yourself when you take care of your health.

Chapter Three

How Your Mind Affects Your Health

The mind is programming, like the software of a computer. It is the storehouse of information of everything that has ever happened to you. Your mind operates through your electrical and nervous systems to connect to every part of your body. Everything the mind does is to help the body survive; to make sure the body is safe, loved and comfortably alive.

What a huge complexity of operations the mind performs in our behalf, all to support our life and learning process. Our mind performs numerous tasks from storing information to instructing our body to "wall-off" toxins (poisons) to protect us. Our mind is a fantastic servant, a controller of our body. It is there to support our lives, not to lead and direct; that is the job of spirit.

Our Mind Helps Us Survive

The mind is a wonderful survival mechanism to help us learn, store and recall information automatically and at will. Our mind runs our human machine with such precision; we do not have to be conscious of its inner functions for it to work. Our mind supports us by storing information that protects us from physical harm and emotional discomfort. We have a built-in alarm system that goes off automatically when there is any possible threat. Have you noticed how quickly the mind goes into action, even when there is no real threat? Have you noticed that sometimes it's as if our "button" has been pushed? This is because of all the data it has at its disposal. Many times similar situations or people can stimulate a response from past events that get linked improperly to our present experience.

Our Mind Can Misjudge Our Experience

A man, who looked like my grandfather, came to visit when I was a child. I ran over to him and hugged him and said, "Grandpa, I didn't know you were coming! I'm so glad you're here!" All of a sudden my family began to laugh as they quickly informed me the man was NOT my grandfather. I ran to the bathroom and hid for the rest of the night.

In the embarrassment of misjudging the person to be my grandfather my mind created some new programming, which turned out to be a benefit: don't be hasty in decision-making. Stop, wait, sense, observe situations, then proceed cautiously. My mind wants to work FOR me to keep me comfortable, not against me causing embarrassing situations. Misjudging can happen, but nothing is ever lost; all can work for our good. So don't worry about making a mistake! We all do. Look for the benefit!

We are Programmed for Protection

The mind judges in order to protect us from all types of hurt or pain. It then responds automatically through the central nervous system to protect us from physical danger, sending up warning signals in the form of feelings held below a conscious level. Pictures come up from the subconscious with a whole library of information to keep us safe physically, comfortable emotionally and "right" mentally.

The Law of the Mind

There are laws that govern the mind. For the mind to survive, it must be RIGHT. So everything the mind does is to be right, proper or justified. This means that in any given moment the mind is acting in our very best interest; acting out of beliefs that keep us protected from harm or embarrassment. You may discover a few minutes later "you weren't right," but the mind does the very best it can with the data it has within its resource center. Sometimes it gets a little hasty in decision-making and has to apologize. This can be embarrassing, so it does not like to make too many decisions. Many times decision-making can be very uncomfortable, the very point the mind likes to avoid. So having the courage to make decisions usually goes beyond the mind, outside of our survival programming, to the source of our being (spirit).

When the mind makes a decision (to be right), it then can create circumstances to prove it is right. It's amazing how the mind can actually filter out any information that would disagree, so you can prove you are right. It's as if something other than yourself is always working to keep you safe and right.

27

The mind functions either in the past or what it believes about the future. It can only act upon the information stored in itself. You are the one who watches your mind. You can notice what is actually true or just a story made up to be right. This requires awareness and letting go of the need to prove you're right.

The Mind Judges out of its Beliefs

Our description of judgment is, "Drawing a conclusion before all of the evidence is in." There is a part of the mind that really thinks, "I know it all." Is it any wonder with all of the evidence it has stored there? The mind can be very dogmatic, having worked so hard for us sorting and storing all that information. The information becomes beliefs and affects our behavior and relationships with others. Judgments come out of those beliefs and then new beliefs form out of judgments. Have you ever wondered why there are so many different, even opposing beliefs? Our beliefs fall into three main categories:

1. Cultural Beliefs
2. Family Beliefs
3. Personal Beliefs

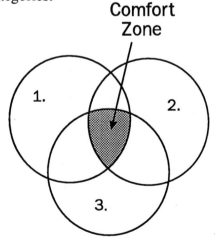

Comfort Zone

Dr. Vernon Woolf shows in his Model of the Mind the way our beliefs overlap and make up our "Comfort Zone." It is helpful to look at the diagram and see how easily we gravitate to this place. Discomfort can keep us from stepping outside this area to look at some other point of view. I call the outside area the "Twilight Zone." It can be frightening to be open to the chance that someone else, who differs from my beliefs, may be right! It can be uncomfortable to go beyond the mind's comfort zone and to be open to another person's point of view. Moreover, the mind cannot tolerate being wrong. It needs to BE RIGHT to survive!

Pause for a moment and put yourself in someone else's place. Look through their eyes at something they believe and you don't. Feel how intimidated your mind is to see another's beliefs without judgment. If you close your eyes, you can image through their eyes better. Really take a look from *their* viewpoint, with their programming, their background, their friends and family. What do you see?

Your Feelings are Signals to Guide You

Feelings of anger are simply your warning system telling you a threat is present. Maybe you're not getting what you want. Anger can mask hurt; it is a signal to stop and look at your situation. Feeling sorry for yourself is just a part of you crying out through a fear that your life is not fair. Your circumstances may need altering. Every message from your mind has survival at its base. Going beyond the negative emotion to the underlying fear, you can appreciate the mind's reactive signal, instead of being controlled by it.

Why Your Mind is Never Satisfied

Your mind functions with programming that it is always needing MORE, BETTER, and DIFFERENT. These feelings affect all parts of your life. They keep you moving forward with your life, but can interfere with contentment in the present moment. Unless you live beyond this programming in the presence of NOW, you function automatically in unrest, always needing more, better, or different. The mind is never satisfied because of fearing any conflict outside its "comfort zone."

On an emotional level as well as the physical level, the mind is programmed to need comfort and a non-disturbed state to survive. If basic needs are not met, a warning signal comes up. Fear is a weapon of the mind to get us to listen. The mind cannot tell the difference between a real or a false threat, so it reacts to ANY possible threat. As you look at your emotions you can go beyond the surface to the underlying cause.

Without Healing Your Emotions, You Do Not Heal Chronic Problems

Stop for a moment. Sense what it feels like to cry or hold tears inside. Do you notice the congestion you feel in the area of your sinuses? Notice how you tense your jaw when angry. Emotions become embedded in the area of the body involved in the sensation and cause a vicious cycle of energy to form there. This can cause emotional blocks to build up that eventually become manifested in the physical body.

I find emotional blocks trapped in the body of every chronic case. I even find people who cannot get rid of allergies, candida or viral infections until the emotions are cleared. If you have a problem that keeps returning, it is a sign of unresolved thoughts and feelings that are now emotional blocks. You can locate buried emotions through muscle response testing (MRT) and can meditate, pray and ask for revelation for your healing. Many times I have asked for the Holy Spirit to guide me in understanding my body and what my body needs to be well.

You can be aware of certain trapped emotions simply by looking at where your body feels blocked or tense. Certain types of emotions consistently cluster in particular parts of the body. Our feelings can help us tune in to our body and expose what needs healing. As an example: self-pity settles in the sinus area and contributes to allergies and sinusitis. Anger settles in the throat along with feeling controlled. Guilt settles in the spleen, pancreas and liver. Feeling unloved affects the heart and lungs. Many more examples are found in the "Manual" and "Reference" books of the Kalos Transformational Healing Series. "Heal Your Body," by Louise Hay also shows lists of ailments that can aid you in finding underlying trapped emotions.

Answering the "Wake-Up" Call

I look at disease as a "wake-up" call to get our attention. Everything the body/mind does is to keep us comfortable and to preserve our lives. A woman came to a Kalos Seminar with a cyst on her uterus. She found out she was holding on to many hurts: blame, anger, resentment and hatred which accumulated in her uterus. Testing her body revealed that she was carrying around unresolved emotions from her past marriage. The hatred for her ex-husband became directed at all men and interfered with other male relationships. What her body was telling her was: she needed to forgive her ex-husband, not for his benefit, but for her own!

When you hold on to experiences that have painful emotions attached, the emotions can contribute to congestion in the physical realm. A situation may happen in which you feel victimized and you do not want to forgive. Your mind feels that person doesn't deserve it. You may say, "I want to forgive this person so I can be well." Yet the heart holds on to old hurts and can't let go. This is where the Kalos Process is so helpful. Sometimes, not until you walk in another person's shoes will your mind and heart transform and let go of the pain. When you look through another's eyes and feel his/her feelings, you then can understand how that person felt right or justified in what was done. Though at the time the person felt justified, moments later the mind may judge differently. The law of life is: we live in what we send out. We will be treated in a similar way we treat others. If you're not being treated the way you want, stop and look at your own actions that could be affecting another's actions. Then start treating others the way you want to be treated. It works!

As the Mind Goes, so Goes the Body

Since the mind controls the body, what it says, goes. If you hold a belief that someone "knows what's right and does wrong anyway," you're not aligned with the natural law of the mind. The breaking of this law creates anger, resentments and stress. All people's actions are directly related to what they think or feel is right, proper or justified in the moment of choice. Their mind can only function this way, no matter how it may appear. A few moments after, they may change their thought and feel guilt. At the time of the action, though, they did the best they could. You can honor your mind's intention to keep you right and justified. You can work with your mind and make allowances for its misjudgments or mistakes.

How the Brain Supports Your Mind

Information is processed through the brain and central nervous system. The brain receives and sends out the information to the appropriate organs, glands, muscles, etc. in the body. Therefore, the brain's communication system has a bearing on the mind's ability to function. If there is a short circuit in the electrical impulses of the central nervous system, information cannot be processed and stored properly. Emotions can switch off or short circuit the communication system of the body. The electrical and nervous systems both send information to the brain.

Our brain is divided into two hemispheres with a hypothalamus gland in between to extract and sort out the information. This gives us the ability to receive, store and give out multi-dimensional data to aid us in decision-making. Every bit of information is used to protect us physically, be right mentally and be safe emotionally.

We Program all Information in at Least Two Ways: How We *Think* About It and How We *Feel* About It

Our two hemispheres in the brain balance our ability to function in a more wholistic way. It is very helpful to see each situation from BOTH – a practical, linear, logical view and also from a feeling, imaginative, creative view. This supports learning easily and relating well to others. Our left brain resolves problems step by step. The right hemisphere sees answers in a flash; it is not concerned with the method of how the answers arrived. They don't even need to make sense. It just is!

Both of these hemispheres are valuable to our mental function and make a contribution to our well-being. It is the functioning of these two hemispheres simultaneously that creates the whole picture and a clear perspective. We are then able to align our thoughts and feelings to bring balance into our life.

Problems Arise When Only One Side of the Brain Can Function at a Time

When both hemispheres of our brain do not function at the same time, blind spots can occur in our ability to understand what is going on. It interferes with our ability to take in, comprehend and give out information in an acceptable form. These blind spots in how we think or feel can cause even more frustration, which makes the problem worse. This "switching off" is called dyslexia. "Switching off" is simply the electrical system to the brain being short circuited to one hemisphere and not being able to function at the same time as the other hemisphere. An emotional trauma, severe injury or illness can cause "switching off." Sometimes a traumatic childbirth experience can trigger this mechanism. I have traced many learning dyslexia problems back to an early traumatic learning experience.

Emotional Dyslexia May be Affecting You Unknowingly

Emotional dyslexia is the inability to use both sides of the brain simultaneously and may be triggered by intense emotions (experienced or denied). You can tell if you are dyslexic in a situation if you become super logical without emotion or over-emotional and illogical. This is not to say that many people are more one way than the other. You are able to tell when you are not yourself. More people than you can imagine "switch off" one side of their brain when confronted with certain emotional problems.

This "switching off" interferes with being able to think straight in intimate relationships or situations requiring important decisions. It can get in the way of acting fully mature around certain people. This is how the term "emotional dyslexia" came into being. Almost everyone has some form of dyslexia, either learning disability or emotionally caused "switching off."

There was a woman, for example, who fell in love with her best friend. It became likely this special friendship would become intimate. As friends, they had wonderful times together. When the chance of intimacy arose, fear came in and literally "blew a fuse!" Her brain began to "switch off" around this person out of the fear that her love would not be accepted. Because of her over-emotional state of fear, she stopped being comfortable around this person. Her deep-rooted fear caused her mind to "switch off" and interfered with her ability to function maturely. As a result, she stopped liking herself around this other person, so they separated. This "switching off" produced a condition of

35

"double-mindedness." She THOUGHT she wanted to be with this person, but FELT she didn't.

Being "Single-Minded" Helps Us Achieve Our Goals

"Switching off" on one side or the other of the brain takes more than will power to correct. I am amazed how quickly we can align both sides when we trace the conflict to its cause. Aligning our mind helps us to complete our goals successfully. When we are "double-minded" we are unstable and move one way then another. We can get close to the results we want, but never actually achieve those results, which can be very frustrating.

An example of this is illustrated in the case of a man who wanted to stop smoking. He was certain he wanted to stop smoking, but never could. In doing a right/left brain test we discovered that he *thought* he wanted to stop, but *felt* he didn't. He was "double-minded" about it. This can happen in any situation. You may think one way about it and feel another. We traced his compulsive feelings back to a time when he tried really hard to stop smoking and his girl friend abandoned him. The discomfort that he felt from his loneliness was relieved by smoking. So now smoking and having a reliable "friend" who wouldn't leave him was connected.

The man saw how his programming had been ruling his life. He committed to using other ways of comforting himself, ways that would not destroy his health. He brought himself to "single-mindedness." Now, by observing his need for comfort, he can take care of it in a mature way and stand by his commitment to health and real happiness.

The Key to Success is – Watch Your Mind

The choices you have made in the past have brought you to where you are today. Most of those choices came out of old programming that began before you even had memory. You can change the old programming and renew your mind. The process is as easy as: listening, choosing, responding and expressing.

Listening – to what you say and how you feel when you are feeling that way (as well as inner guidance).

Choosing – to own your own feelings and thoughts, stop blaming, no one made you feel that way.

Responding (rethinking) – by changing your old thoughts about it, your feelings will change automatically.

Expressing – loving thoughts and actions, based upon God's will for your life and the special way for you to serve.

The mind is programming. It does not think; *we think* and it records. As soon as a thought or experience happens, it becomes a part of our programming. Everything programmed in the mind has already happened (the past) or is an illusion about the future. Spirit functions only in the PRESENT. You were not made to be a puppet for your mind. You were made to live in the presence of spirit, by the presence and for the presence of spirit. We are made as a temple of the living God – Spirit in control, mind recording and body expressing.

The Mind is a Wonderful Servant, but a Terrible Master

It is estimated that most people actually spend very little time functioning in a present-time mode. Most of the time their programming is controlling them. They are on "auto pilot." You can renew your mind by understanding how it works, watching it, and allowing it to be the servant as intended, not a master puppeteer.

You can depend on your mind to act out of programming to automatically keep you safe and alive. You are the one to take charge of new decisions and respond anew to today's circumstances. The mind functions out of decisions from the past that may not be relevant today.

Once the Mind Makes a Decision with Intense Emotion Attached, It Becomes the Rule of Action from that Time Forth

The more emotion attached to decisions made by the mind, the deeper the experience goes. Every experience having a relationship to that decision is colored with it from that time forth. For instance, when I was nine years old my mother died and soon after my father became an alcoholic. Feeling alone and unloved a decision welled up within me: "I am not lovable."

This decision made it difficult for me to accept another's love. I would listen to the words, "I love you," but not believe them. This affected my behavior so much that I was always looking for acceptance and love, because I believed I couldn't be. This kept me *trying* to do what already existed. Little did I realize that other people's love had little to do with me. It had more to do with their own choosing, colored by their decisions made at a young age too. Because of this belief, though, a wonderful benefit evolved: I learned the joy of serving others. As a child, I ran from the fear of "non-acceptance" by compulsively pleasing. Now, as an adult, I am free to choose to serve out of my own love of giving, or notice I am being a compulsive giver.

My mind is always seeking the "freedom from," where in spirit I function out of the "freedom to." How I think about what I do makes a big difference in the level of happiness I experience. Just shifting to "freedom to" from "freedom from" changes my attitude and up-levels my joy. Needing "freedom from" creates compulsions toward compensatory behavior to fill in what is lacking. "Freedom to" is freely walking forward to explore anew. "Freedom to" creates the space for CHOICE to show up.

It Is as You Think!

Thought energy can create reaction just the same as if it were real. The mind does not know the difference between the real and the imagined – the thought and the actual happening. Just thinking of something to which you are allergic can actually cause allergy symptoms to appear. For example, if you are allergic to dog hair, thinking about a dog can change your pulse rate and weaken any muscle in your body.

When any kind of threat is programmed into the mind in the presence of certain foods or smells, etc., an allergy may develop. The mind cannot differentiate between the real threat and the circumstances (food). All gets programmed in as part of the problem.

As an example, a lady came to my workshop allergic to Goldenrod, a flower that blooms in summer. Every time she would go visit her parents she would have to pass a large field of Goldenrods. Each year she would have to put up with that allergy. By going back to when the problem began, she uncovered a very upsetting experience in the presence of Goldenrod. So the Goldenrod got programmed into the upset! By diffusing the upset, her allergy to Goldenrod disappeared.

Not Only Can the Mind Affect Bodily Function, but Also the Body Chemistry Can Affect the State of Mind

An example of how the body chemistry affects the state of the mind is that when blood sugar levels drop below normal, irritating feelings of depression and anxiety can result. These feelings can occur also when the body has a viral or fungal infection. We cannot separate the body from the mind nor the mind from the body. When the body goes into a survival mode with an infection or the blood sugar dropping, anxiety becomes a warning signal that something is wrong. Do not cover your nervous conditions or irritations with drugs; instead heal them. If you want health, listen to your body. Align yourself with the natural or spiritual law that was broken.

Highlights

* Your mind is programming like the software of a computer. Every bit of information is stored from the time of conception.

* Your mind can misjudge your experience, because it brings up all relative information which may or may not be relevant to the situation. It works hard to protect you.

* Your "comfort zone" is made up of your beliefs. Your mind is always migrating back to that zone for protection and peace.

* Your mind is never satisfied. It is always wanting MORE, BETTER or DIFFERENT. Noticing this can aid you in choosing to act out of spirit, which is perfect peace.

* Emotions form out of your thoughts. How you think about something affects your health.

* Pain or discomfort is a "wake-up" call to let you know that something is out of balance. Listen to the call.

* Whatever the mind says – goes. The body follows the directions of the mind, so it works as a barometer for our inner state.

* Information is programmed in at least two ways: (1) How we think about it, and (2) How we feel about it. Having a "double-mind" is when your thoughts and feelings

are not aligned. Every problem has a "double-mind" at its source.

* Problems arise when one side of the brain is "switched off," as in dyslexia. When you become this way around certain people, we call this emotional dyslexia.

* The key to success is to watch your mind. Observing your thoughts and feelings can give you insight and renew your mind.

* You can change your programming by: Listening, Choosing, Responding and Expressing.

* Your mind doesn't think, you think. You are in charge.

* To be in charge requires waking up each moment to choice, living each moment anew. Otherwise you function on "auto pilot," living off of decisions of the past as if they were appropriate today.

* Life is as you THINK. The mind does not know the difference between the thought and the real. Allergic responses can be experienced just by thinking of what you are allergic to.

* Not only can our thoughts affect our bodily function, but also body chemistry can affect our mind. For example, low blood sugar can cause anxious feelings and insecurities to arise.

* If you want health, align yourself to natural laws.

Participant's Page

1. LOOK INSIDE YOURSELF AND IDENTIFY AN AREA OF YOUR LIFE WHERE THERE IS STRUGGLE OR FRUSTRATION – Where your thoughts and feelings are not the same, or where you have opposing thoughts about it. (Example: "I think I want to change my job, but I feel it would be too hard.") YOU CAN USE MUSCLE RESPONSE TESTING, IF YOU KNOW HOW.

2. WRITE DOWN SEVERAL DIFFERENT EXAMPLES OF HOW YOU ENDED UP IN THE SAME FRUSTRATION. (Track your feelings) (Example: "I went to work and my co-worker complained that I was not doing something right." "I went to the club after work and the secretary said I didn't fill out the paper correctly.") The same frustration comes down to "not feeling good enough" each time.

3. WHAT IS YOUR BIGGEST COMPLAINT?
(Example: "Others don't appreciate me, so I am always having to do more to get their approval. I feel frustrated because it seems like whatever I do is never enough.")

4. MAKE A COMMITMENT TO ACHIEVING YOUR FULL POTENTIAL IN A SPECIFIC AREA OF YOUR LIFE. (Example: "I want to be a great partner in my relationship by sharing my deep feelings.")

5. LIST WHAT A FULL POTENTIAL PERSON IS LIKE IN THE ABOVE AREA. (Example: 1. A great listener. 2. Compassionate. 3. Confident.)

Chapter Four

Uncovering Your Hidden Agenda

Every problem has a hidden agenda. The purpose of this book is to open the doors to understanding the major reason for illness, fatigue, depression and every form of suffering. Your mental attitude is the position (or disposition) you take about people or situations, and accounts for the biggest part of your health. There is a hidden agenda that colors your attitude and affects your thoughts and feelings. What is your automatic response when a problem comes up?

I feel that the biggest part of wellness comes from how we interact with life through our attitudes. It is no surprise that two persons can be exposed to a virus, etc., and only one becomes sick. There is a reason some people have an immune system so strong that nothing can break it down, while others falter. There are four major areas that affect our health:

1. Nutrition
2. Exercise and rest

3. Environment (free from polluted air, water, radiation, chemicals, negative people, etc.)
4. Attitude

The first three account for about ten percent of your health each, for a total of 30 percent. They are covered in detail in the Manual. Seventy percent of the factors affecting your health is attributed to attitude. Attitude is the total *subconscious programming relating to your mental/ emotional perspective about life.* More details on this subject are in Chapter Five. Transforming your attitude can bring healing and wholeness.

To be Healed Is to be Whole

Healing comes from the word whole, as does holy. Christ said, "Be whole" to many who were sick. Being whole is functioning in a loving, harmonious, prosperous, healthy state. Being whole is not limited to our spiritual life. It means to be our full potential in every area of our life, as an individual, a mate, a partner in business. Our physical, social, financial and spiritual well-being are a part of wholeness.

One area of your life can be transformed and affect all the other parts. Wholeness permeates all boundaries, because it is about renewing the mind and acquiring new core thoughts about old ways of functioning. It requires looking within yourself for your problems, instead of "out there," and taking responsibility for your life. Give yourself a chance to look through "new glasses." Just pretend that a broken law is at the source of your problem. And you broke the law! Be open to discovering what that is, and see what happens. As you align yourself to natural and spiritual laws your mind renews automatically.

Renewing the mind is the way to wholeness. It is necessary to living your full potential in all areas of your life. If you are discouraged or depressed, your mind needs renewing. If you are not making the kind of income you want, your mind needs renewing. If you are not happy in an intimate relationship, your mind needs renewing. New thoughts result in new feelings about your life. Those feelings affect your attitude. Your attitude is the driving force behind your actions and how you experience your life. AND YOUR ATTITUDE IS AT LEAST SEVENTY PERCENT OF YOUR HEALING PROCESS AND YOUR HEALTH.

As you explore the laws and principles in this book, may you look at your life in a meaningful way and make a commitment to transformational healing. However you cut it, transformation means **change.** It means that you are willing to take a look at what you are doing, when you are doing it, and be **honest.** It means you are ready to open some doors to the unknown part of your life and courageously walk through.

Transform Your Life – Body, Mind and Spirit

The word transformation has taken on many meanings, from Biblical references to pop-psychology clichés.

"Be transformed by the renewing of your mind"

This biblical exhortation is often quoted in relation to:

1) Waking up to your full spiritual potential.

2) Knowing who you are and why you are here on the planet.

3) Carrying out your life purpose successfully.

To me, being transformed means all of this and more, because the mind controls the body. It holds the added meaning of: spiritual, mental, and physical renewal.

Although transformational healing includes an understanding and technology which approaches health in a comprehensive way, this book is only able to cover some of the mental/emotional and spiritual aspects. There is another book in the form of a Manual that is available which covers the physical aspects also. Within its pages you will find ways to understand how your body works and how you can communicate with it on a cellular level. The Manual shows in-depth ways to trace any problem to its cause.

Drawing Distinctions between the Mind and Spirit

It is easy to accept that we are not our body. We use our body. There is widespread evidence to support this. Now, I want to draw some distinctions between the functioning of the mind and spirit.

When the mind tries to imitate the spirit by taking control of your life, it ends up in a deception. The mind can only function out of its conditioned preprogrammed state. Spirit functions in the now.

It is the mind that needs renewing during the transformation process. The mind controls the body. Whatever the mind says, goes. You can renew your mind only by making new choices today. Your old programming cannot renew itself. Your will power cannot renew the mind. Only conscious awareness through the spirit can renew your mind. As your mind renews, your attitude matures.

You can fool yourself into believing you are transformed when you are not, because of the mind's ability to rationalize and justify itself. You can also fall into the pit of judging others and their transformational process. Only YOU (and God) know what is really going on inside you. The tendency is to compare oneself to the worst of others and compare one's mate to the best of others. Comparing can get you into trouble, however you do it.

This book is about getting honest. I feel we transform our lives no faster than we GET HONEST!

Some Steps to Get the Most Results

Pick a project and take it through the following steps. If you do not know what project to use, think of something that really bothers you in someone else, such as an angry attitude or an inability to express deep feelings. Usually the very act that bothers you the most in someone else, is the very thing you are guilty of doing also at even deeper levels. Maybe it's hidden and difficult to see. Maybe it expresses itself in a little different form. If you look deep enough, you will find it.

Allow change to happen; don't "need" it to happen. Struggle is a sign that your mind is controlling, instead of surrendering to the ease of spirit to do the work.

1. Accept yourself the way you are right now (with the problem). You really have done what you could. Be compassionate.

49

2. Own your own programming. Don't blame others (Mom, Dad, boss). Because you own it, you can play with it.

3. Look deep inside yourself to a time when the problem was evident. (This could be a long time ago, or yesterday.)

4. What feelings of frustration, anger, etc. did you have at the time?

5. How often do these feelings come up in your life? What is this telling you about your consistent emotional patterns?

6. Understand your experience. You may want to go to another time when you felt that way. You may want to just be compassionate with yourself for those difficulties. (Be willing to look at any pertinent information that will help you understand why you began having that attitude.)

7. Allow compassion to well up within you for yourself and others with the same problem. (Compassion has an element of forgiveness in it, for others as well as yourself.)

It is Only the Truth that Sets Us Free

It is my hope that you will want to take time to look into your own life and answer the questions on the Participant's Pages. Please take the time to do this. It is when you become quiet and meditative that you hear the Spirit speak and discover hidden knowledge. My most enlightening times have been when I have been alone, many times while studying. I stopped and looked inside. Seeing the truth (what's so) still sets us free. It doesn't take struggle. It can happen by just seeing a hidden agenda – like turning on a light in a dark room and noticing the intricacies of what's there.

I remember a story about a man who awoke one dark night to realize that a thief was climbing in his window. All the owner had to do was to turn on the light and it frightened the thief away. Deceptions work in the darkness, while Truth loves the light. Transforming your life may be uncomfortable, but not painful.

Transformation Can Be as Easy as Turning on Lights and Looking at What Is Really There. Are You Willing to Take a Look?

Since the mind has a need to be right, it will immediately align itself to truth. This begins a domino effect supporting rapid healing.

Look at the cause of your complaints, so problems don't return (in this or another form).

You can spend too much time chasing symptoms around, never getting to the cause. Too many people experience a beautiful healing – that does not last. The symptom was temporarily treated, but the cause was not discovered and healed. Therefore, it was a temporary relief. When we heal the cause, the symptoms disappear – permanently. Every problem has a cause. Every cause has a cure.

Highlights

* Every problem has a hidden agenda. An underlying pattern of beliefs brought you to where you are today.

* There are four areas of your life that are affecting your health:

1. Nutrition
2. Exercise and Rest
3. Environment
4. Attitude

* Your attitude has the biggest effect on your optimum health and success in life, affecting about seventy percent of your healing process.

* THOUGHTS and FEELINGS which you may not be in touch with make up your attitude.

* Feelings are thoughts put into action. They are a result of beliefs or justifications for beliefs.

* Every problem has a cause. Most of the time there is ONE MAJOR BELIEF AT THE CORE OF YOUR PROBLEM. You just keep playing the same tapes and repeating the same pattern!

* You transform your life by the renewing of your mind. Understanding the distinctions of the body, mind and spirit can help you to take charge of your attitude.

* You can notice whether you are expressing your life through the mind or spirit. The mind functions only in the

past (programmed) state and spirit functions only in the now.

* You can take the opportunity to involve yourself in a program to support your healing the underlying cause.

* You can uncover the hidden agenda that is controlling your life. I challenge you to participate now!

* Transformation can be as easy as turning on lights and looking at what is there. Seeing the truth (what's so) can set you free!

* When you heal the cause, the symptoms disappear – permanently.

Participant's Page

As you discover your patterns of behavior, you can choose to go beyond them and make new choices that support your happiness. Be honest with each question. Be still and contemplate each answer. Usually the first thought or response that comes to your mind is the most accurate.

1. IN WHAT AREA OF YOUR LIFE ARE YOU SUF-FERING THE MOST?
(Example: "My emotions – I get overwhelmed with frustration which turns to anger and affects my relationship with my mate, children," etc.)

2. WHAT DO YOU WANT TO HAPPEN THAT IS NOT HAPPENING?
(Example: "I want to relax, enjoy my relationships and stop being angry with my family.")

3. HOW LONG HAS THIS BEEN A PROBLEM?
If this problem dates back to when you were very young, you may need some assistance. So use something that is recent.
(Example: "Since I got married," etc.)

4. WHAT CIRCUMSTANCES WERE GOING ON IN YOUR LIFE AT THAT TIME?
Who was involved? Where did you live and how did you **act**? Write all the details down clearly. (Example: "My marriage was decided so quickly, I didn't have enough time to prepare. I was overwhelmed with too many tasks to finish

before the wedding date, because of moving, so I was exhausted.")

5. HOW DID YOU FEEL ABOUT IT?
(Example: "I felt frustrated, pressured and controlled.")

6. THIS WAS PROBABLY NOT THE FIRST TIME YOU FELT THIS WAY. NOTICE ANY PATTERN OF FEEL-INGS OR BEHAVIOR FROM AN EARLIER TIME.
(Example: "I was really frustrated in a previous relation-ship. It seemed that no matter what I did, I was wrong. I did a lot of work on myself and the relationship still failed. My needs were never met. I was hurt deeply.")

7. WHAT WAS YOUR BIGGEST COMPLAINT AT THE TIME? NOTICE IF IT IS SIMILAR TO THE PRESENT TIME.
(Example: "I worked very hard to please her and didn't have my own needs satisfied. This caused much frustration, WHICH IS MY PRESENT-TIME PROBLEM!")

After you identify a pattern, continue to the next chapter and identify your PERPETUAL ATTITUDE! Every one of us has a subconscious-driven attitude that colors our experiences in life. It is this attitude that is the biggest factor in how we process information. When you learn to watch this inner programming, instead of being tossed around by it, you will have new skills to renew your mind.

Chapter Five

Your Attitude Is Showing!

Your attitude is by far the biggest factor determining your health and happiness.

Someone once said: "Our attitude determines our altitude." I feel much closer to God when in a great attitude. I can look at what is going right or what appears wrong. Both have value, depending on the circumstances and both have their consequences. Some people will get over one ailment, just to get something else. Their attitude brings them back to where they began.

Your Attitude Comes from Subconscious Conditioning

Your attitude is formed out of your feelings. If your prime attitude is feeling not good enough, you require others to give you praise and appreciation. However, not receiving praise and appreciation can make you feel depressed or angry; you get to be right about not being good enough. On the other hand, if you feel good about yourself, your attitude meets situations with a sense of value. Your attitude can con you into believing things that aren't true.

I remember when I was very young, I would pretend there were angels or fairies watching me. They would check out the work I was doing. It gave me great pleasure to do a good job, because of being noticed allegedly by them. This contributed to my having a happy attitude about working. My family was not the type that gave much recognition, so I created my own. I still remember how excitedly I would finish a job and feel really good about myself, as my unseen partners would applaud me. My attitude was, "others are watching and appreciate the good job I do." My attitude of being watched over, had nothing to do with someone else being there, it had to do with my own made-up programming. When my mother died, Jesus became my unseen partner. For many years I felt watched over. Even today, I never feel alone.

Your Attitude is Dependent upon Your Thoughts

Your thoughts control your attitude. It is empowering to know that only YOU are in charge of your thoughts, since no one can think for you. Although others can influence your thoughts, you rule in this domain whether you realize it or not.

The most heroic attitude I have ever encountered was Reverend Wurmbrand's. This man spent fourteen years in a Communist concentration camp in Poland. His body bears deep scars from being tortured. Two different times he spent six months in solitary confinement. Bread and water was his existence. And yet he recalls that in that dark cell he praised and worshipped God and rejoiced in the Love of Christ. He reports that Christ visited him there. He lived in what he radiated out – love. It was his loving attitude that got him through those dark years and then out into the mission field again.

Feelings are thoughts put into action.

Your attitude wells up out of your subconscious mind, forming out of your feelings, will and emotions. Feelings are a result of thoughts and can be changed by changing your thoughts. You can change your thoughts by *choice*. Emotions result when feelings are judged by the mind, whether positive or negative.

You can release unwanted emotions by uncovering the hidden judgments. Judging creates fuel for your attitude and motivates you toward goals. It can also stop you from reaching a goal.

The power is within each of us to choose at any time what we want to think. I can determine if I am living out of Light by my attitude, as well as if I am living out of a deception (negative emotions). It gives me a barometer to see the truth (what's so) about my life.

We have the Power to Change Our Attitude

To transform your attitude is to transform your life. You transform your life no faster than you are willing to be honest about it. Don't get stuck in the reasons why your life isn't working. Get in touch with your bottom-line state of being – your attitude. You may be creating a life to prove you are right about being a failure, rather than being happy or successful.

Ask yourself: "How happy am I?" Through awareness you can observe your attitude and CHANGE your THOUGHTS.

Thoughts are enlivening or destructive. You can choose to focus on that which is beautiful, supportive and of good report or you can focus on what is missing. It is up to you, because only you can choose your thoughts.

Feelings are merely thoughts put into action and make up your attitude. You are in charge of the conversation that goes on inside your mind. You can watch this conversation at any time. What do you think about when you do not need to think of anything? Do your thoughts bring enthusiasm into your life, or doubt? Are you in a state of appreciation or are you defensive, looking for ways to prove you are right? You can change your attitude by changing your thoughts. You can shift your mental habits into seeing benefits, instead of horror stories.

Seeing Benefits Can Change Your Attitude

I rejoice in knowing that whatever happens in my life works a benefit. No matter how it looks on the surface, I can count on it to be helpful. Spirit has taught me to look for the benefit in everything. I live in the faith that God cares and wants me to succeed continually. This is easier to do as I surrender my will. An attitude of gratitude is a great attitude!

You can experiment with the possibility there IS a benefit to EVERY situation. Look for the benefit. You will find what you are looking for, consciously or unconsciously. If you are looking for disappointment, you'll find it. If you look for rejection, you will find that. As you look for love, you find an abundance all around you. Notice how much more love you experience when you are sending love out!

Expressing Love Can Change Your Attitude

We cannot feel love coming toward us; only as we send it out do we enjoy its warmth. If you want to experience what I'm talking about, stop for a moment for an experiment as you read.

Focus your thoughts by going back to a time when you were a young teenager deeply in love with someone who didn't love you. You felt so excited every time you thought of this person. Your heart throbbed. You really felt "in love," but they acted as if you didn't even exist! Now, think of a time when someone really loved you, but you didn't want them. You didn't want anything to do with this person. Did you feel their love coming toward you? Of course not, all you felt was repulsion. We live in what we send out. Love is only experienced as we give it.

So if your attitude could use some sprucing up, I challenge you to find a new way to express love dynamically in the world. You can begin by "being there" when you're there. For me "being there" is the most basic form of loving. Without it, love is mechanical and more of a doing than a being. Being there and looking right into a person's eyes gets their attention. Being there is just that: being present with them and their being. Without getting someone's attention, it is difficult to express the love you are. Patiently, you can wait for them to be with you too.

Try it! Try reaching out and touching people more. Expressing love through touch can bring bonding and caring to a deeper level. When you are untouchable, people sense

61

indifference in your attitude. Sometimes a hand shake and smile can turn a stranger into a friend. There are so many ways to love. Start contemplating on ways to open up and share the love you are.

Notice how a child reaches out spontaneously, not concerned about what others think. Notice how quickly the child forgives. Maybe this is what life is about, a continuum of loving and forgiving.

Living Your Purpose Blesses Your Attitude

There is joy in knowing you are living your life's purpose. It promotes a superb, positive attitude. I am not speaking of making positive affirmations about your life, which are not true, so don't last. It is not negative to see the truth of difficult circumstances when we see those circumstances as a positive challenge with an inevitable benefit. What I am saying is that you can BE the space of a positive attitude no matter how tough life appears. Being the space of a positive attitude means that you are willing to watch your busy mind instead of being run by it. Your mind can leave you feeling at the effect of life, rather than at the cause.

You can choose to relax and be an active observer of the benefits involved. Living your purpose connects you with the knowing that whatever happens, you will see an ultimate benefit. Remember the story of Reverend Wurmbrand in the concentration camp.

You can quickly develop a positive attitude once you know who you are in relation to a loving God and your Life Purpose.

You will rejoice as you manifest that purpose in the world. Nothing is so exhilarating as knowing that you are always in the right place at the right time. When your life is about your purpose, it becomes so much bigger than the little incidents that happen along the way – the little happenings that the mind can make so important.

When your eyes are on the "Big Picture," you keep your life in perspective to what is really valuable. You then can overlook the mundane and look for the long term benefit.

Highlights

* Your attitude is the greatest determinate of your energy level and health.

* Your attitude is your natural way of handling situations and comes from your subconscious mind.

* Your attitude is not primarily dependent upon what others think, but what you think about yourself.

* Your attitude forms out of your feelings, will and emotions.

* You can observe your attitude and up-level your thoughts. It is your thoughts that create whether you feel comfortable or uncomfortable.

* You can shift your thoughts easily by looking at the benefit in each situation. You can train your mind to shift automatically by habitually catching yourself in your horror story.

* Then be grateful! An attitude of gratitude is a GREAT ATTITUDE.

* Express more love in your life. Reach out to more people. Be there, touch, and express more loving thoughts to them.

* Living your Purpose blesses your attitude with enthusiasm and joy. You can be the space of a positive attitude no matter how tough life appears.

Participant's Page

ATTITUDE CHECK LIST: BE HONEST!

(Always - 10 points, Never - 0, or any number in between)

1. I awake with a smile and look forward to my day.

2. I appreciate who I am.

3. I love myself and others consistently.

4. I am not swayed easily into negative outlooks or thoughts.

5. My life is full of meaning and purpose.

6. I am free to feel my feelings and express them properly.

7. When problems arise, I meet them as a challenge.

8. I see a benefit in everything that happens to me.

9. I quietly say, "Thank you, Lord," many times a day.

10. Others like to be around me, because I am seldom depressed.

11. I easily see good in ALL others.

12. I encourage others to own and appreciate every experience.

13. I listen to my inner guidance and act on it.

14. I am refreshed by loving thoughts frequently during the day.

15. I smile frequently, even when no one is around.

16. I have a good sense of humor.

17. I love my life and know that God loves me.

18. I appreciate the beauty around me often throughout the day.

19. I notice the thoughtful things that others do around me.

20. I can laugh at myself easily.

ADD YOUR POINTS:
    180 to 200 - Excellent!
    160 to 179 - Good, but needs improvement.
    140 to 159 - You are really hard on yourself.
    120 to 139 - You're running on negative emotions.
    100 to 119 - Your programming is running you.
    Under 100 - Crisis situation, get help NOW!

Chapter Six

Why You Act the Way You Do!

What Our Common Programming is and the Effect it has on Everything We Do

The following model of how the mind becomes programmed for survival is useful in understanding why we act the way we do. The model includes seven basic decisions and shows us how fear comes into being. These seven decisions are our core programming that affects everything we do. These decisions cause an automatic chain of responses for physical survival by warning us of any danger. They support our comfort by warning us of possible threats to our emotional and physical safety. What a wonderful built-in support system!

I find it fascinating to watch my mind function through these Seven Basic Decisions. I get to watch my thoughts move between wanting my own way and wanting to please. "Mind watching" empowers me to move into the neutral zone of CHOICE, instead of being driven by my programming. When I become defensive, I know I'm functioning from these old basic decisions. I can then "rethink" the situation and make a meaningful choice.

Our Core Programming – the Seven Basic Decisions

The first six decisions were made on a subconscious level before we ever knew what was going on. They formed out of our experiences that had deep emotional attachment. Anytime a decision is made with great emotion attached, it becomes the rule of action from that time forth. It becomes core programming. Every decision that follows is tainted by the one before it. It's as if these hidden decisions control our behavior. And they do, when we are functioning out of programming, instead of WHO we are.

These decisions are beliefs about how life is. Out of these implicit decisions we, as children, decide what action needs to be taken to be right, proper and justified. They prescribe what we unconsciously think we need to make our world safe and secure.

The succession of the first six decisions spans from birth to the preteens and they are made on a subconscious level. The Seventh Decision is made consciously at a critical time in a child's life, a time when feeling important is needed to build a secure ego. The following story is not meant to be taken as unalterable fact, but as a general guide to understanding how your mind works.

The Story of How We Got Programmed

Before we were born, we enjoyed a beautiful floating state in the womb. There was warmth and protection there. Everything we needed to survive was provided. Then the day came to be welcomed into the world. What a celebration!

First Decision

After squeezing through a very small opening, so small that our head comes out shaped like a football, we are greeted into a cold room. Then someone sticks some object down our throat that makes us choke! (Of course, the well-meaning doctor is only trying to clear the air passage by removing any mucous so we can breathe.)

If we are not yet crying, we are spanked until we do (crying expands our lungs to breathe)! What a welcome! Is it any wonder that at birth we make a decision with great emotion attached to it, that:

1. "Pain is bad, comfort is good. The purpose of living is to be non-disturbed."

To add to the discomfort some relative might exclaim, "Oh no, it's a girl!" or "How ugly, what a strange looking creature that is." It is astonishing how many people think they were not wanted at birth or were the wrong sex.

The pain and discomfort at birth makes it VERY IMPORTANT to be NON-DISTURBED.

Any time a decision is made with great emotion, it becomes the basis for all other decisions.

69

Looking at the FIRST DECISION: "Pain is bad." Is it true? From a realistic view with more information than the little child had, we know that pain is not bad. In fact, we would probably self-destruct before the age of five if it were not for pain. Pain is really our friend, not the enemy it was programmed to be. Pain exists for our survival. Without pain we could burn or injure our body beyond repair. PAIN HELPS US SURVIVE.

Pain can be experienced physically or emotionally. The mind creates feelings of emergency out of beliefs of being threatened. Emotionally, we must feel loved to feel safe. Survival depends on our feelings of comfort. This comfort programming is so embedded in us that unless a baby is held and loved, it cannot assimilate calcium to grow and survive. Feeling loved affects the parathyroid gland which metabolizes calcium. Unless we feel accepted, it is difficult to maintain a desire to live. My own father told me just weeks before he died that he didn't have a reason to live. This had nothing to do with what was actually so, it was simply what his troubled mind felt as it ran his life.

This First Decision that the purpose of living is to be non-disturbed creates a FALSE purpose in the mind, stating COMFORT to be our main motive. Is this true? Is comfort our major purpose to be alive? Comfort is a form of survival, not a fullness of JOY. We all have a divine purpose for living which most of the time is not comfort-able, but causes us to stretch. And stretching may hurt! We are here to learn and grow. And most of our growth comes out of uncomfortable experiences!

This NEED to be comfortable could be our only prob-lem!

70

ALL problems could very well be based upon this ONE, because all following decisions are influenced by it.

The fear of becoming uncomfortable becomes our prime directive.

The result of this need to be comfortable is that FEAR comes into being. The fear of being uncomfortable! The mind, in its fear of disturbance or discomfort, sends out many signals to warn us. These signals come in the form of thoughts and feelings. Emotionally the mind is afraid of rejection. Intellectually the mind is afraid of being wrong. Physically the mind is afraid of injury. All are forms of pain. This programming is wonderful for survival, but terrible if it rules our lives. When we run FROM a problem or discomfort, instead of moving TO a divine CHOICE (in the moment), our lives can end up in a constant survival mode. This survival mode initiates fears and compulsions which are acted out in various forms.

Second Decision

The SECOND DECISION is based upon the first decision. Having it VITAL to be non-disturbed, it then becomes VERY IMPORTANT. At a moment of need or pain the young baby makes the next critical decision:

2. "It is important to be non-disturbed, so I must have my own way NOW!" (And by complaining loud enough, I get it.)

An infant complains if its needs aren't met right at that very moment! A child does not understand what it means to wait. It only knows what it NEEDS NOW. This self-centered behavior is valuable for survival, but can be very obnoxious if found controlling an adult.

This is an important decision that lets others know of a need. The baby cries for food, for diaper changing or for some other basic need cared for. There is nothing wrong with having our own way. In an adult it's only a problem when it CONTROLS one's life. As we mature, we can change those needs to preferences; but functioning out of programmed survival, the young child has no choice. This child programming is still in us.

Third Decision

Between the age of one and two, a new kind of conflict comes into a child's life. Up until this point it has been fed, held and cared for whenever it complained enough. The day finally comes when the child doesn't get what it wants. Mom or Dad says, "No!" For example, Junior wants to eat when it is only fifteen minutes before dinner. He has always eaten when hungry. Mother decides he is now big enough to eat with the family. She does not give in to Junior's reaching out and complaining for food. She wants him to wait and eat in a few minutes. Junior doesn't know how to wait! He has always received what he has wanted, when he wanted it. So mother leaves the kitchen and Junior climbs on a chair and gets into the cookie jar.

Functioning from the programming that pain is bad and comfort is good and the purpose of living is to be non-disturbed, he doesn't think twice about doing what he wants to satisfy his hunger. Then mother returns and catches her son in the act of disobedience for the very first time. Taking the cookie and slapping Junior's hand is very painful, physically and emotionally! A NEW DECISION is in order! The earlier decision is no longer working. He ends up feeling very disturbed!

Based upon the previous decisions and made with INTENSE EMOTION attached to it, the mind makes its THIRD DECREE:

3. "It is important to PLEASE others, to be non-disturbed."

For the first time in Junior's life conflicting desires enter his programming. He now must choose whether to "have his own way" or to "please others."

Conflict between our thoughts and feelings can cause a tug - of - war to go on in the mind. Part of us wants to go one direction and part of us to go in another. This is what inner struggle is all about. As we grow we work at balancing these two parts. Every problem we have will go back to a kind of "double-mindedness." We sometimes have two opposing thoughts, but most of the time our struggle is with feeling one way and thinking another. When aligned, life becomes easier and more harmonious. Usually, we make several painful attempts at having our own way before letting go to become a pleaser. This decision begins with pleasing Mom and Dad, then goes beyond the home to pleasing authorities.

Fourth Decision

The FOURTH DECISION is made about the age of four or five. It supports you with rules and standards for your young life. As the child surrenders to authorities of all kinds, the day comes when a discovery is made. If you do as you are told and the AUTHORITY is wrong, it's not your fault! You are SAFE and beyond blame! Hence, the next decision:

4. "It is important to do as I am told by my authorities to be non-disturbed."

Another interesting response comes when the mind discovers: "Since I was doing what you told me to do, I am not responsible for my actions." This makes one feel even more safe. So Junior begins to appreciate being part of a group or belief system, where all the rules are clear. Keeping the LAW gives a feeling of safety and confidence and support. Living by the rules gives a child a sense of satisfaction and accomplishment. It expands the area of comfort and safety to a social level beyond the home.

It is comforting to know that whoever is in charge knows what is right and wrong and how you can stay non-disturbed (right). It provides standards to live by, so we can feel safe socially. Wouldn't it be terrible if there were no rules?

What about traffic rules? How would you like to drive without any lanes and arrive at a corner the same time as twenty other cars not knowing who was to go first? So rules keep us SAFE and create the space for civilization to function in a harmonious way. In fact, maybe without this decision civilization could not even exist!

The next Decision builds strongly on Decision Four. Along with needing to please authorities and the law, a strong need develops to please peers also. Peers begin playing an important role in a child's life.

Fifth Decision

5. "It is important that I be different (so I can be accepted)."

The need to be different comes from a feeling of not being enough just as one is. A driven need for acceptance motivates this decision.

Changing to "fit in" becomes a major motivation in a child's life about the age of eight to ten. Now it becomes IMPORTANT to do whatever is necessary to please peers, even if it means changing some part of yourself or your appearance. Making the FIFTH DECISION of being different adapts the child to his environment. To make and keep friends is very important at this age. A child may become very emotional if he feels he does not "fit in." When we bring this decision into adulthood without being balanced with decision number six, it can cause us to wonder who we are. We can even become obsessed with compulsory pleasing. Some extreme reactions to this decision include acting out a martyr role. In the martyr role you can lose touch with who you really are.

I remember an incident that happened in my mid-teens while out on a date. My new friend and I were driving along the Hollywood Freeway in Los Angeles, when I asked him how he wanted me to act. His reply startled me and made a profound impression. He said, "Just act yourself!" I blanked out because I didn't know who that was. Being raised in different foster homes and with different stepmothers, I was used to acting however others wanted me to. I just wanted to "fit in." This began a profound search to find out who and what I really was.

Sixth Decision

The SIXTH DECISION is made after coming to the conclusion "I can't be different; I've got to be ME!" Pleasing others has run its course and the child becomes more independent in his thinking. He stops wondering who he is and starts feeling more important. Though he may not be sure who he is, he is sure he is not the person others think he is. The individuation process takes hold as he stops his compulsive pleasing to meet another's expectations. So the sixth decision is made with great emotion again, based on the NEED TO BE COMFORTABLE and be himself.

6. "It is important that YOU be different." "If you want US to get along, YOU will have to change! You will have to accept me the way I am. I've gotta be me!"

This decision may look rebellious in nature, but it's only the personality exerting itself to bring balance and fairness. After years of pleasing to be comfortable and needing acceptance the day comes when you MUST be whatever you want. This causes a drastic change in the personality, depending on how important it was to please. Emotionalism and overreacting may appear in any situation. Frustration and guilt can come from not being able to please and also have what you want. Many times anger comes from feeling you can't be who you want to be, have your needs met and still be accepted. Stress is the result.

This Sixth Decision moves you back to the anger side of the personality, which is usually not the norm since around the age of two or three.

The "I need to be me" side of the personality may come across as selfish or domineering to the extreme. Anger can redevelop to rule your world, just like it may have done as a young child. By tuning out emotions you run your life from the logical side of the brain. This is not to say pleasers are not logical. Pleasing may be the most logical thing to do at times. Since anger is such an intense emotion though, the mind has to build a big wall to cover it. The building of this wall makes it difficult for ANY emotions to get through. Walls are ways of protecting oneself from deep hurts. Deep hurts covered by anger will always have something to do with not having one's "own way" or life not being fair.

As you can see by the following diagram, the pleaser side of the personality experiences fear and guilt – fear of not pleasing or guilt from NOT doing something they felt they should. Chronic pleasers can in turn become very resentful when they initially feel unappreciated.

PICTURE OF MAN/WOMAN

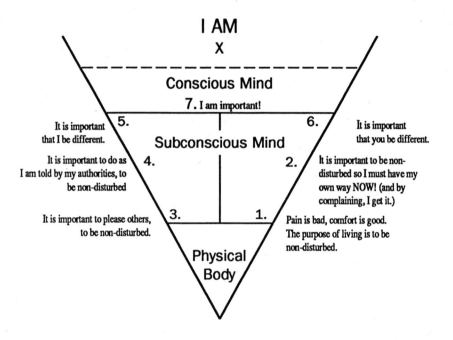

I AM
X

Conscious Mind

7. I am important!

5.   It is important that I be different.

It is important to do as I am told by my authorities, to be non-disturbed

It is important to please others, to be non-disturbed.

Subconscious Mind

6.   It is important that you be different.

2.   It is important to be non-disturbed so I must have my own way NOW! (and by complaining, I get it.)

1.   Pain is bad, comfort is good. The purpose of living is to be non-disturbed.

Physical Body

4.

3.

There is a catch to being a pleaser. The catch is they unknowingly must get something out of the deal. Without it being an even trade, hidden resentment causes either physical illness or unusual behavior. The pleaser personality usually manifests the most ailments, due to the resentments that build up from not being appreciated.

Pleasers can also feel guilty when they don't do anything to justify that guilt. They just believe they should do something! How do you feel when someone you know needs help and you don't give it to them? A pleaser can actually suffer with emotional pain that interferes with digestion, elimination and hormone production. The entire endocrine system may also become affected. Hence, pleasers have more chronic illnesses.

Guilt and its accompanying resentment is probably the biggest destroyer in the body – most dangerous when concealed.

This flipping from pleasing to having one's own way causes fluctuations in temperament. The left brain, or logical mind, then learns how to think emotions, instead of feeling them. An accumulation of emotions can build because of not sharing them. Then these suppressed feelings cause fear of what would result from this big dam being broken. Closing down the sharing of feelings builds frustration and stress, thus making the next decision imminent.

These first six decisions are made on a subconscious level. The conscious mind is unaware of their presence. You can observe your own and others' behavior through these decisions, simply by acknowledging they are there. I find them extremely helpful in working with people, because they expose core programming and blind spots about themselves. And I can watch my own mind!

Seventh Decision

Usually by the age of twelve the SEVENTH DECISION is made. This decision comes at a very crucial time in a child's life – puberty. The individuation process is in full effect and this decision is valuable to further healthy development.

7. "I AM IMPORTANT"

Proclaiming this to the world brings bottled up emotional energy to the surface. It usually comes with, "So you'd better listen to me!" This is a healthy decision, as one can then know that one is balancing their self-esteem. One needs this to grow happily into maturity. Self-esteem is of utmost importance for a healthy mature attitude and part of the individuation process of the maturing ego. It is the very foundation needed for later successes. A healthy ego is able to surrender itself to serving God and others. Without a strong ego there is little to surrender to something greater than ourselves.

Understanding This Process Helps Our Children Grow Happily

This basic decision can create a generation gap if the parents do not understand. Teenagers need their thoughts and ideas listened to. They need the same respect that is expected of them. When treated like irresponsible children, they usually rebel. Allowing them to make more of their own decisions is helpful. This is a conscious process they are aware of. By this time they can understand the consequences of their behavior. Encouraging them to be responsible and take care of themselves (physically, mentally, emotionally, and spiritually) supports this decision in a mature way. Above all LISTEN TO YOUR CHILDREN!

Children will usually live up to the image you give them of themselves.

Imparting positive thoughts are valuable when a child is developing. "If a child lives with criticism, he learns to condemn." Children mimic the people around them. They look to adults to find out how to express themselves maturely. They need models of mature self-esteem at this age. Many adults are still functioning in programming from their childhood, because they did not make a strong enough statement to the world, "I am important." Some adults act like little children in big bodies. They have not developed in the area of self-esteem. Instead, they live from insecurities that prevented them from making a strong statement about their value. Living out of past-time emotions triggered by present-time events can result in feelings of unworthiness and shame. Most problems in life stem from deep hurt feelings that project "there is something wrong with me."

Old Decisions from the Past can Affect Us Today

When a pattern is set at a certain age, it becomes a way to deal with similar problems when older. All the programming comes up when triggered by a like situation. The old tapes play.

For example, Sheryl was frightened by a dog who bit her at the age of three. Though she is now forty-five, she is still afraid of dogs. When around dogs she breaks out in a sweat and her heart races. These are the same responses that came up when she was a child. Because of this response, she developed an allergy to dogs. Once there is *understanding* why the physical response is there (and the present situation is not the same), the mind can create a new, more mature response to the situation. Instead of Sheryl becoming three years old in the presence of dogs, she can now respond as an adult. Many other simple allergies are relieved quickly. Understanding is the key. As the truth is seen we are set free!

I challenge you to explore these concepts with me and see if they fit your experience also. I love working with people and hearing their stories. I love to see them discover the truth that sets them free of sickness and upsets. By understanding how your mind works you can be a masterful OBSERVER and take charge of your programming. You can correct your scripts and renew your mind.

Remember, YOU CAN'T RESOLVE PROBLEMS USING THESE DECISIONS OF THE MIND. YOU CAN ONLY SEE HOW THEY AFFECT YOUR LIFE. They are the substance with which problems are made. Your problems are only going to be resolved when you go beyond the programming to WHO you are instead of acting like a robot that automatically needs to please or needs to have your own way. You can RETHINK every situation and act upon inner spiritual guidance.

You are not your programming. You are spirit, created in the image of God with all the attributes of God. It is plainly seen that the above programmed mind is valuable, but not joyously happy. Your mind would prefer being safe or right than to be happy. It is up to you to choose happiness. It is up to you to choose to follow Spirit's inner guidance in each moment, now and now and now. Choice functions beyond the mind. Choice is your birthright. You can choose to or not to at any time. You can renew your mind to support your happiness as well. Choice is of the spirit, while deciding is of the mind. The mind decides based upon the programming there.

Your purpose for living is NOT just to be comfortable. Some of my greatest accomplishments were not comfortable. It is when I have done something uncomfortable (that I didn't want to do), that I have learned the most and stretched the most. I feel the best about myself when I have gone through that which I feared. Joy results, not from resisting discomfort, but by choosing to follow the Spirit's newly guided way.

The Unresolvable Problem

The one big problem in all our programming is "unresolvable;" however, we can make it disappear. Through the "Picture of Man," we can see how *the mind* developed with a false purpose for living.

Because every other decision the mind makes is an extension of this first false decision, a BIG PROBLEM is created. In addition, that problem is unresolvable!

Every person who has made the decision "Pain is bad, comfort is good and the purpose for living is to be non-disturbed" has this same problem.

It is unresolvable in the respect that it is core programming of the mind. It is very valuable programming to help our bodies survive, but interferes with a happy, productive life.

The big problem comes in when this subconscious programming rules our mental and emotional states. We all want comfort, but:

Needing to feel comfortable to take action in our life is like the tail wagging the dog. It draws us into a wasteland of insecurities and fears with a mirage of never ending false hopes.

Perhaps sometime in the future we will no longer need that kind of programming. However, for this moment the mind is in the survival mode, so we need to understand how to deal with it.

Even though this big problem is unresolvable, we can create the space for it to disappear.

We (spirit) can be the MASTER of our MIND. Observing how this problem shows up in our lives will give us the power to go beyond it, since the problem is unresolvable.

Taking charge of your mind begins with AWARENESS: Watch the mind. What are your deep-felt emotions and reactions to other people's behavior? Notice where you are coming from at any time. Be honest about where you are and where you want to be. Through seeing your true feelings without resistance, you can go beyond the one big problem. It's that easy!

If you are feeling angry or afraid of rejection, you can *choose* to love yourself and care for yourself in that moment. This *choice* will open a door for you to go on to support your highest good, then love others and live your purpose fully.

Sometimes *you* need to be the one to do what you want someone else to do — love yourself!

These basic decisions operate our minds. Watch them as they affect your feelings and decision-making. Notice which side of the personality is your comfort zone – Pleaser (fear/resentment) or Own Way (anger). Though each one of us has both sides, we can gain marvelous insight into our lives by noticing where we are at any given moment. Then we can act maturely out of a new choice!

Our programming functions out of a need to be comfortable, a need to have our own way, a need to please, a need for rules, a need for love and acceptance. We are all programmed this way. All of these decisions are living inside us. They help us to survive. Without this programming we would have self-destructed early in life, so appreciate it! We all move through these seven basic decisions continually, none of which resolves problems.

In conclusion, there is only ONE problem: OUR NEED TO BE COMFORTABLE. This is bottom-line programming based upon a false purpose for living. Though it is unresolvable, we can create the space for it to disappear. We can pause and watch our mind. We can renew our mind to support our joy and stop resisting discomfort by *CHOICE*.

We can choose to care for ourselves, commit to other people's happiness, then act out of those commitments (learning as we go) and BE the space of Love.

Highlights

* Pain is bad, comfort is good. The purpose of living is to be non-disturbed. (Survival-based programming – beginning at birth.)

All of the following decisions are based upon this decision, which is false, but creates the bottom-line survival programming for our benefit.

* It is important to be non-disturbed, so I must have my own way NOW! By complaining loud enough, I can get it. (Anger based programming.)

* It is important to PLEASE others to be non-disturbed. (Fear/Guilt based programming.)

* It is important to do as I am told by my authorities to be non-disturbed. (This is a common ground for people who like to use authority to prove they are "right.")

* It is important that I be different (so I can be accepted). (Fear/guilt programming.)

* It is important that YOU be different.
If you want US to get along, YOU will have to change! You will have to accept me the way I am.
(Anger based programming.)

* I am important! So you better listen to me!
(Ego based programming.)

Participant's Page

1. WHICH OF THE SEVEN BASIC DECISIONS MEN-TIONED ABOVE DO YOU MIGRATE TO MOST OF THE TIME? (Example: "I usually am the one to please the other person, rather than need to have my own way.")

2. GO TO A TIME WHEN YOU LIVED OUT OF THE OTHER SIDE OF THE SPECTRUM. (Example: If you are a pleaser, go to a time when you wanted to have your own way.) Notice how you felt. What was the uncomfortable feeling you wanted to stay away from? Through identifying your "comfort zone," you can look more clearly at your thought patterns. These patterns are not good or bad. They are simply your way of functioning. When you understand how you function, you will then make allowances for yourself and access the compassion you deserve.

3. NAME YOUR PRESENT MAJOR "DISCOMFORT ZONE."
(Example: Working in a job where people are unfair, relationship, etc.)

4. WHAT IS THE PROBLEM (DISCOMFORT) YOU ARE RUNNING AWAY FROM RIGHT NOW? (Example: "I don't want to look for a new job. I don't like being turned down.")

5. IS THIS PROBLEM (DISCOMFORT) AFFECTING YOUR DECISION-MAKING IN RELATION TO NEW OPPORTUNITIES IN YOUR LIFE? (Example: Just staying in the same old rut.)

6. IS THIS PROBLEM (DISCOMFORT) INTERFERING WITH YOUR ABILITY TO EXPRESS HOW YOU FEEL? HOW?

7. IS THIS PROBLEM (DISCOMFORT) MAKING IT DIFFICULT TO ACCOMPLISH YOUR GOALS. HOW?

8. DOES IT SOMETIMES FEEL LIKE SOMEONE OR SOMETHING IS CONTROLLING YOU, RATHER THAN WHAT IS IN YOUR BEST INTEREST?

9. HOW OFTEN DO THESE SAME FEELINGS COME UP?

10. WHAT CAN YOU DO TO REMEMBER TO STOP, PRAY, RETHINK AND ACT IN YOUR FULL POTENTIAL?

You can renew your ability to achieve your goals by RETHINKING your experience. You can seek inner guidance from the Spirit to open doors. You can own your feelings and be free to experience them, even though they are uncomfortable. You can have a happy life.

Chapter Seven

The Vicious Cycle

The Body Responds to the Warning Signals of the Mind

The "sick cycle" is the body's response to any possible threat or stress. When we were very young, an automatic defense system was set up to preserve our lives. If we perceive a threat, even if it isn't an actual threat, the body reacts as if we were in danger.

When we perceive something as a threat, a signal goes out through the nervous system to prepare the body to run or fight. Every activity carried on by the body is to preserve the very life of the body. The Sympathetic Nervous System is on guard to pump adrenalin into the blood to run faster or fight the foe ferociously!

The body's response system works automatically, not knowing it is sometimes functioning under a false threat. The mind does not know the difference between what is real or unreal. The mind believes anything disturbing its comfort is a threat. We perceive physical pain as one of the threats to our body's survival. Emotional pain is also seen as a threat to our feeling loved and accepted.

There are many feelings that threaten the body/mind. Feeling unwanted is a threat with which many children grow up with. We have gone back in processes where some discover they were not wanted by one of their parents. I have not found this to be the case with both parents. Some students have experienced their mother's attempt to abort them. This leaves deep patterns of insecurity in the psyche. Also, the inability of parents to express their love openly promotes an immature pattern of being unlovable.

The sick cycle is a vicious cycle that increases the loudness of our body's message. If the cycle is understood, it can enable us to identify and diffuse any threats. The more understanding we have about our body and its responses, the more support our mind gives us to be well.

The following diagram explains what is going on at a cellular level when one perceives a threat to the body/mind. All the senses of the body are part of an alert system to warn the mind of danger.

When a threat occurs, the mind immediately reacts with an interpretation, which starts a chemical reaction in the body.

The chemical reaction expressed through cellular activity or unusual behavior goes on until the vicious cycle is broken. The healing arts are designed to break the vicious sick cycle. Psychiatry breaks into the cycle after unusual behavior occurs. The medical world breaks into the cycle after cellular activity shows up in the form of an ailment.

You can break into this cycle immediately after the first response, by correctly interpreting the event. You can identify what is true, rather than buying into false feelings of emergency. You can stop the cycle right here!

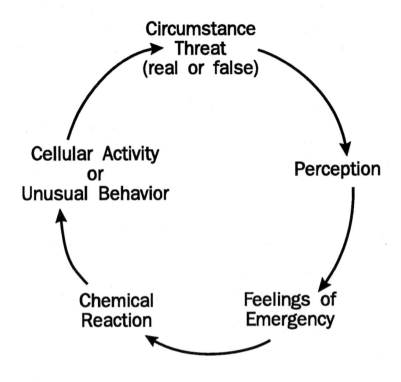

There is a Cellular Response to the Perceived Threat

1. False feelings of emergency arise with a perceived threat.
2. The mind responds with a chemical reaction to protect you.

3. Cellular activity or unusual behavior is the result of this chemical reaction. The body compensates and adjusts.
4. Imbalances occur out of the chemical change that takes place that can create physical ailments. Unusual behavior can pave the way to mental or emotional ailments.
5. The problem itself creates another threat to the body, which gets interpreted again. And on the vicious cycle goes.

The Cycle's Downward Spiral Can be Stopped

The faulty perception that created the response to the false threat can be changed. This changes the effect upon our body. *When the mind thinks or feels that it has made a mistake, it quickly goes to work to make everything right again.*

This is why healing can take place immediately or quickly after what I call a "Kalos Process." I have seen growths disappear rapidly. I have seen people miraculously lose unwanted weight right after a Process and the body's organs come to normal function.

Once we had a doctor come to our Seminar and take a blood sample of one of the participants. This person had been ill for quite some time with a viral and fungal infection in her body. She had very low energy and could hardly make it up her stairs at home. He let the class see the blood under a 1400 power microscope and pointed out the toxins and conditions that showed up there. After this person did a Kalos Process, which cleared emotional blocks and early childhood programming, the blood was tested again. It was exciting to see her body had already gone to work and turned on the part of the immune system that had not been working before. As a result, the massive infection had disappeared.

Our magnificently designed body comes with an extraordinary repair shop. By being aware of what is a real threat and not reacting to false threats, you can intervene in the sick cycle and reclaim your healthy birthright. This is a valuable part of renewing your mind and making a big difference in your health and happiness.

We can break into the cycle through conscious awareness and process out any deception immediately. We can then keep in balance and prevent false interpretations, to help prevent unwanted cellular activity or unusual behavior.

What is a Real Threat?

You may be asking now, "What is a REAL threat?" An example of a real threat is to open the door where you work and have a big, snarling bear growl in your face. The sight of the bear causes the adrenalin to pour into your bloodstream. This gives you an enormous amount of energy to run faster than you have ever run before or to fight the bear. The problem is that when you feel threatened by your employer, your mate, or someone else, your body reacts with the same adrenalin flow. It responds as if it were REAL.

If you are feeling like running away from any person or part of your life, this adrenalin seeps continually into your system. It can make you very toxic.

93

Our Para-Sympathetic Nervous System is Inhibited when Threatened

Another problem arises out of false feelings of emergency. When you're living with feelings that your acceptance or comfort is threatened, your para-sympathetic nervous system does not turn on to digest your food. This para-sympathetic nervous system also governs the production of hormones and sexual drive. When you are in a possible threat, or afraid one will arise, the body cannot produce the needed enzymes and hormones. Instead, it maintains an "on guard" stance.

Tension blocks the circulation and proper energy flows in the body. Your mental state even affects the way you breathe. Holding one's breath particularly affects the oxygen level within the blood stream and does not allow the necessary flow of energy to replenish the body's needs.

Identifying whether or not you are facing a real or a false threat can make a difference in your health. Relaxing and doing your best gives yourself a chance to watch without reacting.

You can use your breath to slow down, stop, center yourself and prepare yourself to observe your life more closely. Being still, breathing, listening to inner guidance and linking the feelings with the past will help you take charge of intercepting this vicious cycle. You then can uncover the truth quickly and easily.

"Know the Truth and the Truth Will Make You Free"

If the real cause of this cycle is not taken care of, resentment builds up and blocks inner guidance. Unless I can "see the truth," I am not free. It can be discouraging to make allowances, breathe and listen to inner guidance and have this pattern come back again. This has happened to me when I felt I was not understood.

When emotions have built up inside of me, it is usually because of experiencing something outside of what I think "should" be. When I "should" on myself or someone else, I am really saying, "I know all about it, so you can't teach me anything." Expectations arise out of thinking we already know, when we don't. "Shoulds" set us up for failure every time. Expectations can be devastating when we place much importance on them. You might ask, "What about the things that really ARE important?" Yes, there are important aspects to our lives, but the mind places importance on everything that might affect our comfort.

The next time an upset happens, notice the rationale concerning what the mind has decided. Is there a threat linked to its origin? Surprisingly, you may find the programming driving you relates to an incident of the past and is not even relative to what is happening today.

For example, when someone raises a voice at me, I find I feel like a child again. I then must go within to check my true feelings. Anger triggers my little child programming that occurred when my father yelled at me. Following his anger, I usually got hit, mostly along the side of my head. These fears became attached to any angry or raised voice. My life was ruled by the fear that I wasn't accepted. Then

I feared I wasn't worthy of love and couldn't measure up to my Dad's expectations.

These fears also became attached to my experience of male energy. My little child programming comes up when I am with an angry male. When my mind rules me, I can even become dyslexic and prove I am as weak and incapable as a child. My mind gets to be right as I lose another battle of empowerment and sink into a deep need to feel loved. However, now that I am seeing the link between what IS real and my programming, I am released from remaining in these false threats.

Understanding the Origins of Our Compensatory Behaviors

Some people use food, alcohol, television, sex, or one of many compensatory behaviors to comfort themselves. I am the type who cannot eat when upset. I have gone several days without eating because of emotional upsets. When the body/mind feels threatened the defense mechanisms come in to relieve the stress and bring comfort. This is one of the biggest causes of over-eating and sexual promiscuity. The mind wants to compensate for the discomfort, even if it means punishing you for not "being enough." There is a war going on in any perceived threat, whether it is real or false, inside or outside.

Seeing the Benefit of Whatever Happens

By looking for the benefit in each experience, I can move from reaction to calmness more quickly. Just going through the process of choosing to see the benefit, my attitude changes.

I once was teaching a Seminar when a very embarrassing situation arose. It was my first time to teach "How the Mind Works." During the Seminar, I used some confrontation techniques thinking this would accomplish the goals of the workshop faster. It was an experience I shall always remember. I doubt that the other person will ever forget it either. For me it was an initiation in "Being free to experience whatever comes up." While I was speaking, a woman stood up and said she did not agree with what I was saying and was leaving immediately. She went on to attack much of what the Seminar was about. I felt a hot wave go down from my head and bathe my body. I'm sure I must have turned several shades of red. As soon as I was aware of feeling embarrassment, I felt free to experience what was going on. As quickly as I experienced the feelings without resistance, my body relaxed and gratitude came in. This only took a few seconds. Looking for the benefit then came easy.

The woman did leave, but called after the workshop and apologized for her behavior. She said she had received much benefit from being there and even greater benefit by seeing herself running away. Running was what she did all her life. She realized that any time she would get uncomfortable in a situation she would leave. The Seminar gave her the opportunity to observe her behavior in a safe but dynamic way. She came back to the next workshop to learn more.

97

Sometimes we might not know the benefit right away. It may take a long time to see the value of the incident that happened. Therefore, why wait to understand? You can accept the principle by trusting Life to bring up the perfect situation. Doing this helps me give thanks in all situations.

We can have Fun Going Beyond the Mind's Story and Get to the Cause

It becomes *clear while observing the sick cycle, that whatever we resist persists.* By allowing all circumstances to show up in your life without resistance, though uncomfortable, puts you in charge. It is so wonderful to know that we don't have to DO anything. Usually just terminating a behavior will bring balance into our lives. Anyway, let's face it, there is no way to go back and prove positively that anything would have been better if it were done differently. So have fun getting honest with your upsets by linking them to their real CAUSE.

Highlights

* The body has an automatic defense system to protect us from danger.

* The mind does not know the difference between a false threat and a real one.

* The body goes through a series of effects when it believes there is danger. This causes cellular activity in the form of chemical imbalance (physical illness) or unusual behavior (mental illness).

* You can break into this vicious cycle quickly through conscious awareness and find the hidden deception.

* Seeing a benefit to whatever is going on can move you to peace quickly and easily. It is also valuable for breaking into the "vicious cycle."

* Trust life to bring up the perfect situations for you.

Participant's Page

1. LONG TERM AILMENTS HAVE A VICIOUS CYCLE GOING ON.

We invite you to take a look at your own experience of life and see if you have a vicious cycle going on. We invite you to identify whether it is a real or false threat. Most of the time it is a false feeling of emergency. When the cause is identified, link it back to when it began. If it began before the age of memory, a Kalos Process will assist you. If not, you can use your own inner focus and replay some of the old tapes.

2. HOW MANY TIMES IN THE LAST WEEK DID YOU JUMP TO CONCLUSIONS TOO QUICKLY. WHEN YOU FIND YOURSELF IN A VICIOUS CYCLE, WHAT METHOD DO YOU WANT TO USE TO WAKE YOURSELF UP? ALL COMPULSIVE BEHAVIOR HAS THIS VICIOUS CYCLE GOING ON.

It will help you to have a pre-assigned behavior to switch to automatically when an upset happens. (Examples: Recite a special quote or scripture, STOP and breathe ten times, close your eyes and relax, pray, etc.)

3. RETHINK YOUR INTENTION TO SUPPORT YOUR SUCCESS.

Make sure your priorities are clear. Recommit to your health and success. Re-examine your purpose for living and assign the proper time to fulfill it.

Chapter Eight

Renewing Your Mind

The Key to Exploring a Happy Life

This book is a journey, this chapter an exploration. You can explore new possibilities for a happy life by experimenting with the techniques described here. You can enjoy this journey to the extent that you apply its methods. Only you can make a difference in the quality of your life. God already is sending you love, light and blessings continually. You can stop and drink of the Spirit's Essence or ignore the abundance of opportunity around you.

Chances are you have some people around you who really care about you and your well-being. They would love to see you really happy, not only for their benefit, but also for your very own joy in living. Can you imagine how much God wants your happiness also?

Your journey will take you to a path of least resistance.

It is amazing how quickly discomfort leaves when it is not resisted. Resistance caused by fear perpetuates stress in your life. If you will "let go" of your resistance and experience your experiences, feel your feelings as they come up, discomfort won't last. You will find that what you feared was only a little twinge in the stomach or a warm feeling in your head. The giants you think are there are not after you! It is only your mind resisting the discomforts in life to keep you safe and alive. You only have one problem. It's unresolvable, but you can create the space for it to disappear through not resisting it. Just experience any discomfort in the moment. You can even thank it for protecting you and then let it go. When I say, let it go, I mean don't resist it, but experience it so fully that it is no longer feared. Notice if it feels warm or cold, dark or light, big or small, round or sharp. Get into what the feeling is really feeling.

Are you willing to listen to your mind – listen to the conversation that goes on continually inside you? Have you ever felt "embarrassed to death?" Have you thought that someone was a "pain in the neck?" Notice your internal conversation. What are you always complaining about? What are the words you constantly think of on a daily basis? Are they coupled with fear or filled with faith?

Only you can be in charge of your mind. Your mind is a wonderful servant because it helps you survive, but a terrible master because it functions from programming of the past. That programming may not be relevant to what is happening right now. Your mind needs updating and renewing. You can **learn to RETHINK your experience** by being present to the new situation, now!

Are you willing to experiment?

The following will help you understand how to rethink each new experience. It is my hope that you will open to the possibility that you are much more than you ever dreamed. You are spirit, created in the image of an understanding, loving God.

Understanding Who You Are

Our body/mind/spirit is so well integrated that it is sometimes difficult to understand where one part begins and the other ends. It is easy to forget that we are more than a body, but also a living soul.

Though our body may be destructible, we are not. We are an eternal and forever BEING. *We are human beings, with a body and with a mind.* You program your mind and your mind controls your body. The body is the form, like the hardware of a computer. The mind is the software with all the bits of information stored there. Spirit is life; the essence of our Being. Without such, there would be no life in the body.

So we **have** a body and we **have** a mind. We are not what we have. We are created in the image of God with all the attributes of God. We have all the potential that children have to be like their parents. We are an infusion of Love, Joy, Peace, Kindness and Patience expressing out through CHOICE.

Our mind functions out of emotions and logic while focusing its attention on what it needs to keep comfortable. This is not CHOICE, this is survival. What has happened in the past may not be the same as the present situation, so our programming may not serve us fully. We need to rethink what is going on in the light of new information. This is simply to stop and notice our thoughts and feelings and whether they are aligned with our intentions. Many times we have a wonderful intention, only to express it so immaturely that no one can get the positive motive at its source.

If you will go back in time and look at your own life, you will see that whatever you did had a positive intent behind it. It may not have been "the highest good," but somehow you justified it or actually felt you were right. Even justified actions have justice behind them and so operate out of positive intents.

Since the mind takes such a strong position about being right, it is intimidated easily. It becomes defensive and anxious. The only way to go beyond its automatic response is to stop, look and rethink the situation in new light. This requires consciousness – the presence of spirit. (I use a small "s" to describe our spirit and a capital "S" to describe God's Spirit. I am not saying the two is not or cannot merge into one. I am only using this as a distinction for understanding.)

What helps me transform my life is my consciousness of Spirit, there to be my guiding light, there to renew my thinking process from survival to truth. Knowing that God is always there to count on, gives me the courage to explore the truth. I love to ask for direction and follow, as my mind surrenders to the will of the Spirit. I get to see miracles happen. My mind renews in the present moment of now, as I see the truth through spirit. I can replace old fears with a new creation based on a harmless world, knowing I am loved and supported.

Our Mind Renews by Surrendering to Spirit

To transform your life out of survival programming requires TRUSTING SPIRITUAL GUIDANCE. You can stop at any moment and look within for understanding and guidance. You can ask and receive. It doesn't have to be done in a special way, just be receptive.

Invite the Holy Spirit in to take over and guide you; then trust the prompting you receive. You will know when you are directed by Spirit, because a beautiful peace will take the place of your anxious mind. Even though you may feel uncomfortable in carrying out your inner directions, there will be a light shining your way, assisting you in rethinking the situation.

The following is a story of trusting inner guidance:
I was praying one morning on what God wanted me to do that day. As I meditated, the answer came to go visit a certain sick lady I heard about a few days before. I only knew she was in bed most of the time with severe migraine headaches and went to the hospital every week for pain shots.

As I got up and prepared to leave, my stomach began to feel queasy. I felt really embarrassed to tell this lady that God sent me to help her. I was young in the healing arts and insecure about sharing my art. I especially felt embarrassed to tell her that God wanted me to see her. My mind was resistant, but my spirit was willing.

I left home with the hope that my weird feelings would leave me. As I approached her house, a rush of resistance made me feel like turning around and leaving. I *surrendered my fears to God and kept walking*. When she came to the door in her robe I introduced myself and unexpectedly blurted out, "God wanted me to come to see you."

She smiled and invited me in. We had a wonderful visit. As soon as I was inside and sharing with her about what might be causing her migraines I felt peaceful. She agreed to follow the dietary program I suggested. I arrived a stranger and left a friend. I received a letter from her a few weeks later saying that she had followed my advice and had been free of headaches. She stated, "I just returned from a trip without a headache and without a box of candy." Her appreciation came in several letters to follow.

The joy in my heart was much greater than the awful feelings of embarrassment. And my mind got another chance to renew itself, to LOVE and TRUST God.

Renewing the mind is not a one time situation. It is an ongoing event moment to moment. There is no magic button to push to change your bottom-line programming forever. There is only remembering WHO you are without resistance, and the TRUTH of your experience. Your need to be comfortable will stay there to give you many chances to surrender to Spirit.

When the mind is a humble servant, the war stops within and we experience a Love that rejuvenates and regenerates our body. When living "in spirit" the aging process seems to slow down or stop. I have even seen it reverse itself.

When I live from a spiritual source, I am grateful for every experience, knowing that a benefit is about to appear! I am constantly amazed at how much God loves me and cares for my welfare. It inspires me to go on and keep trusting.

A beautiful peaceful balance takes place as: Spirit directs, will obeys, mind records and body carries out. In this format of functioning you will discover more happiness than you ever thought possible. You are called to live a life of joy and success.

"Do not be conformed to this world, but be transformed by the renewing of your minds, so that you may discern what is the will of God – what is good and acceptable and perfect." Romans 12:2.

Highlights

* You deserve a happy life. You were created to have an abundance of joy. You were told to RENEW your mind! It was created in a way for you to survive from being a young child to growing into adulthood.

* Your mind functions out of programmed experiences of the past, basing its information on what will keep you safe and comfortable. It is always wanting you to be right, proper or justified. Appreciate it!

* You can renew your mind by surrendering to Spirit. When the mind is a humble servant to Spirit, the war stops within and you will experience a kind of love that rejuvenates and regenerates your body. When living "in spirit" the aging process seems to slow down, stop, or reverse itself.

* You program your mind consciously and subconsciously, then your mind controls your body. Without connection with Spirit your mind runs solely on programmed responses of the past, which are tainted with judgments which may have nothing to do with the present situation.

* Rethinking your experience in the Now allows Spirit to BE in charge of your life. Spirit functions only in the NOW, while your mind functions only in the past (which you can't change) or what it thinks about the future (which is an illusion).

* Living each moment from a new CHOICE (of the spirit) transforms old problems with fears, anxieties, doubts and

petty irritations into challenging events that bring a joyful life.

*   I can learn to look for the benefit in any situation to transform my attitude and watch how much God loves and directs my life.

*   A beautiful, peaceful balance comes into your life as Spirit directs, will obeys, mind records and body carries out.

Participant's Page

PRACTICE THESE FIVE STEPS TO RENEWING YOUR MIND. TO TRANSFORM MEANS TO SHIFT YOUR THINKING OUTSIDE THE CURRENT PATTERNS. YOU CAN TRANSFORM YOUR LIFE BY THE RENEWING OF YOUR MIND, AS YOU:

1. WATCH YOUR MIND. NOTICE YOUR THOUGHTS AND FEELINGS. IF YOU ARE FEELING IN LESS THAN A LOVING OR PEACEFUL STATE, IT MEANS YOU ARE IN A DECEPTION (BELIEVING A LIE).

2. STOP, OBSERVE, OWN YOUR FEELINGS. DON'T BLAME SOMEONE ELSE FOR FEELING THE WAY YOU DO. YOUR FEELINGS WERE TRIGGERED FROM EARLIER EXPERIENCES, PROBABLY YOUR YOUTH. DON'T TRY TO CHANGE THEM, BUT SEEK TO UNDERSTAND THEM. SUCH AS, "I FEEL THIS WAY BECAUSE I WANT TO BE UNDERSTOOD" ... ETC. (YOU MAY WANT TO IDENTIFY WHEN IT BEGAN.)

3. RETHINK THE SITUATION. LOOK AT YOUR POSITIVE INTENT. WHAT IS IT YOU REALLY WANT OR THINK YOU NEED? USE COMPASSION.

4. ASK GOD FOR A WAY TO EXPRESS WHAT YOU WANT IN A MATURE WAY AND SPEAK IT ALOUD. NEW POSITIVE THOUGHTS WILL COME FORWARD TO SUPPORT YOU.

5. SUBMIT TO GOD'S INNER GUIDANCE. AS YOU SURRENDER THE WAY OF THE MIND (TO BE RIGHT) TO THE WAY OF THE SPIRIT (LOVE AND COMPASSION) A CHANGE HAPPENS! FREEDOM FROM THE NEGATIVE FEELING MAKES WAY FOR TRUE PEACE AND HARMONY TO ARISE. IT'S A HAPPENING!

In the next few chapters you will be given some specific methods for renewing your mind on even deeper levels. As your awareness increases, you can identify the perpetrations (lies) that creep into your experience. You will be able to identify emotional patterns that have been with you most of your life and transform them into mature action. You can learn the "Perpetration Game" and catch yourself in your programming.

Chapter Nine

Making a Garden of Your Life (By Weeding Out the Three C's)

There are three "C's" that cause unwanted disharmony in your life. They are in opposition to natural laws, so they bring upsets wherever they go. The three C's keep you stuck in an emotional and judgmental state that causes repercussions in those around you, while concealing the beautiful essence of who you really are. They are like weeds that choke out the wonderful seeds of love, harmony and peace that make up your spiritual nature.

You can create a heavenly garden of your life by eliminating these three C's:

1. Criticizing
2. Complaining
3. Condemning

Someone once said: *"There is only one thing more contagious than enthusiasm–and that is un-enthusiasm."*

An attitude of criticism that constantly complains about what is missing or what should be different can grow like a cancer within a family or a business. The negative contagious energy flows like shadows over all who meet it. It can be so subtle you don't even realize its presence. Sometimes you get so used to it, you forget how damaging it is on your attitude. You can get sucked into its flow and end up not liking yourself, while "shoulding" on everyone else. I'm not saying we always live in a floral scented atmosphere where negative emotions do not even exist. What I mean is: How we look at our world directly affects how we respond to it. IMAGES get programmed into our mind, colored by our attitude.

Though you get stuck by a thorn when you pick up a rose, you can appreciate the beauty of it without complaining. It is time to realize the benefits of the thorns and appreciate the protection they give the rose; without such they wouldn't exist. It is out of seeing the benefits in life that your attitude transforms.

You experience Life out of the very energy you give out.

If you want to live in love, give out love. It you want to live in beauty, give out beauty. If you want to live in appreciation and gratitude, be appreciative and grateful. You live in what you radiate. You wither in what you try to bring toward yourself. The very act of needing to bring it toward yourself is saying that you don't have it! Maybe most of your unhappiness is the result of your complaining that you need to be happy.

Life is an inside-out event. Appearances can be deceiving. Having is a result of, not a reason to. Life springs forth from the inner realm of INTENTION, the design of your will.

What are your intentions for your Life?

Stop, think, what kind of a garden do you want to create around you? You get to choose your life of actions. For every action there is a reaction. There is no one to judge (even God reserves that for after death). There are only actions and consequences. You can choose what you want. You prepare the soil of your life through intentions by your will. You plant seeds through the grace of your spirit by your faith. You water your garden with loving thoughts and actions.

It is up to you whether your faith be positive or negative. "A good tree brings forth good fruit." At any time, you can look at what is going on and find out what you've planted. Look at the fruits of what you have. Just take a look at what is working and what is not. If you are having a difficult time discerning this, ask your closest friend or a parent. They love you the most and will be honest with you about how they see your life. I remember the first time I asked God to let me see myself the way He sees me. It was a shocking experience, but gratifying to make the needed shifts in my life.

You are the designer, gardener and harvester of your Life. Each person has free will. Aligning yourself to natural laws and God's plan for you makes living a whole lot easier.

CRITICISM, COMPLAINING, CONDEMNING ALL
CHOKE OUT AND DESTROY YOUR SELF-ESTEEM,
PEACE AND JOY.

Two Things to Forget
(While Working and Playing in Your Garden)

There are two things in life to forget! I mean really
forget! Remembering them can only cause you much grief.
I experimented with this priceless advice at the young age
of twenty. It has been an inspiration to me throughout many
years.

Some may think it silly or too simple. Yet in simplicity,
I have found the basis of creating the proper soil for Peace
in a stressful world. I can still remember sitting in a
classroom of adults while the teacher shared the two things
to forget in life for happiness. I didn't realize at the time
that they could help me turn my stressful life around. These
two rules prepared the soil of my heart to receive the seed
God wanted to plant within me – His Love.

1. Forget everything good I do for others.

This admonition changed my life, as my pleaser role
sought for approval and fairness that didn't exist. My mind
was always doing for the reward in it. I was always needing
others' approval – always looking for acceptance to feed my
insecure child within.

Applying this advice turned my frustrated world around
and gave me a new look at how I was living my life. Trying
to please others, especially God, was all for approval. It
was my "little child" programming. Feeling unwanted, as a

child, created a need in me to do all that I could to please others to be accepted. The "I can't say no" syndrome became a compulsion that ruled my life. This resulted in overwhelming frustration from becoming too busy and never being able to please enough. Then, I would resent not being appreciated for ALL I had done. Fabricating all this stress kept my attitude under attack and criticism at my door.

When you get needy for another's approval or appreciation, stop and look at your motivation. Let go of the false need for approval and move on. Letting go of "what others do that you don't like and what you do for others" allows you to meet each situation anew. The Spirit can then enter spontaneously and create a new frame of reference in which to live. Most of your old programming was placed there by a little child just trying to survive. By the age of two much of your programming was set; by the age of six about eighty percent is in place. After our teens, change becomes more difficult.

2. Forget everything bad anyone does to me.

This means in the moment, as well as whatever has happened in the past. If you find you can't forgive and forget, take it through a Kalos Process and heal it. (See Book Two, Kalos Transformational Healing Series.) Don't let resentment choke out and destroy your peaceful state.

After collecting this storehouse of beliefs as a child, you spend the rest of your life acting out of those experiences. I am amazed how powerfully our mind can create evidence to prove it is right. Until our mind renews with new experiences, we keep repeating the same old programming, time after time.

How We See Something Creates Our Experience of It

We Experience What We Believe
Then We Believe What We've Experienced

MAYBE . . . We can look at our world at a distance or up close and it wouldn't matter. Much of what we experience is because we expect it to be that way. Therefore, it is our attitude that must shift for our experience of life to change.

We can expand possibilities in our lives by experimenting more with our true experience of it versus what we once expected it to be. Is that possible? *Maybe we can only see through the programming inside.* Aligning yourself to a perpetual positive attitude creates positive actions around you.

Shifting Your Attitude May Align Your Life

Science has corroborated the following hypothesis through the sub-atomic building blocks of life. In quantum physics the particle and the wave are what make up matter. The appearance can change depending on how you test it to be. If you use the test to determine if it's a wave, it tests to be a wave. If you use the test to determine if it's a particle, it is a particle.

Maybe our experience of life is like testing for a particle or a wave. Life may only be whatever we expect or look for it to be.

Maybe the mind works in the same way and adapts to any experience, depending on the programming it has about similar experiences. Understanding this stops me from judging "my viewpoint" as being the "only" viewpoint. It opens me to the possibility that other people's experiences are as valid as mine. It creates the space for: "Believeth all things."

We can make a difference in our lives by living in the PRESENT EXPERIENCE of the way it is, rather than our belief about it. Living in the presence of NOW helps me experience oneness, while my beliefs keep me separate. Everyone seems to believe differently in most areas. Even people of the same family or same organization have different beliefs. There is a way we can experience more oneness in our life and less separation. Love is the primary force that holds all things together. We can use UNDER-STANDING instead of judgment. We can open to the possibility that others too are living out of their programming of the past, which to them is right, proper or justified. We can tell the degree our mind is renewed by how much oneness or separation is experienced moment to moment.

Experiencing Oneness or Separation

ALL LIFE'S EXPERIENCES ARE FLOWING ONE WAY OR THE OTHER: INTO ONENESS OR SEPARATION. (Notice how oneness feels like heaven and separation feels like hell.)

If I'm happy, I'm in gratitude and experience oneness.

When feeling troubled about anything, my mind will go looking for someone or something to blame and create separation.

When I blame myself, I create separation from myself.
When I blame someone else, I create separation from them.

Separation is like the illusion of death. The body dies, but the soul lives on. Maybe we ARE part of a whole, otherwise we could not experience oneness in the first place. Whatever we experience as separate from us in any way, may be the very part of us screaming out for healing. Maybe we can use the very obnoxious acts of others to tell us what we need to heal in ourselves, because there is nothing separate from ourselves and nothing to prove except to ourselves. Just holding this, not believing it, can assist you in transforming your life.

The very part of you that fears separation, yet creates it, is your mind. Your mind functions in duality for survival, your spirit in oneness. Your life changes when you live out of the "new moment" of the spirit. Your mind renews each moment you are living "in the now," instead of the old programming based upon needs to survive. The mind is motivated by needs, yet you are spirit.

Notice, right now you have no needs. Everything in this moment is provided. You have enough air to breathe and sustenance to live. Everything else is your choice. This very moment you can be aware that all your needs are satisfied. Your wants can be taken care of in time. Wants are intentions, they are not needs. Getting honest to what is ACTUALLY going on right now will remove you out of your struggle to survive and bring you to choice where the magic takes place. Renewal happens when you align with spirit in the now. Is your mind racing ahead, worrying about "if your needs will be satisfied in the future?" When your mind starts worrying just notice that you are in a mental robot mode. Then, choose to move back into BEING in spirit. As a human BEING, you are always in the power of choice. As you "choose to," instead of "*run from,*" you will be preparing the soil for a beautiful life. Much of what you want to change in your life is on a conscious level with a subconscious cause. Usually, programming changes more easily by releasing it through going back to the time of its origin. Here a Kalos Process will work best.

Only you can plant your garden, nurture it to grow and remove the weeds that get in the way. Only you can make choices that create results for your life. I invite you to experiment with first: weeding out the three C's and second: forgetting the good you do for others and the bad they do to you. When you do this the spirit of oneness flows up out of your heart and spills into the lives around you – what a blessing!

Highlights

* You can make a beautiful garden of your life by weeding out the three C's: Criticizing, Complaining, and Condemning.

* Criticizing, complaining, and condemning break natural laws of the mind.

* You experience life from the very energy you give out. If you give out complaints, your life is about complaining. If you give out love, it's about love. You live in what you radiate.

* There are two things to forget: everything good you do for others and everything bad they do to you.

* How we see something, creates our experience of it. We see through the programming inside.

* In quantum physics the particle and the wave become whatever they are tested to be. They take on the characteristics of the intention of the test.

* Your attitude can determine much of how you experience life. When you look for the positive, the positive happens.

* Looking for the benefits in life can support a positive attitude. Knowing that everything is working for your good brings peace and contentment.

* We are constantly experiencing oneness or separation. When we are aware of what energy is present, an empowering experience can follow. We can choose to be conscious of the heavenly state of love, peace, oneness, thus blessing our lives and those around us.

* You are in charge of your life. You can rethink any situation and make new choices. It is Spirit that renews the mind.

Participant's Page

1. FOR THE NEXT WEEK KEEP A RECORD OF HOW MANY TIMES YOU USE ANY OF THE THREE C'S. I MEAN ACTUALLY TO WRITE IT DOWN ON A PIECE OF PAPER OR BUY A MECHANICAL HAND COUNTER. NOTICE IF CRITICISM COMES UP MORE AT HOME OR AT THE OFFICE. WHAT MAKES THE DIFFERENCE? WHAT METHOD WORKS FOR YOU TO CHANGE THIS HABIT? USE IT!

2. NOTICE HOW LONG IT TAKES YOU TO MOVE FROM A NEGATIVE TO A SUPPORTIVE ATTITUDE. YOU MAY WANT TO RECORD THIS TOO. YOU WILL FIND THE LENGTH OF TIME YOU NEED TO SHIFT SHORTENS DRAMATICALLY.

3. FOR THE NEXT THREE WEEKS WATCH HOW MANY TIMES YOU BLAME SOMEONE OR SOMETHING FOR YOUR PROBLEM. STOP, RETHINK THE SITUATION, OWN THAT YOU CREATED IT, AND SHIFT INTO A "RESPONSIBLE" MODE.

4. CHOOSE TO BE HAPPY! NOTICE HOW OFTEN YOU HAVE THAT CHOICE. IT PRESENTS ITSELF CONSTANTLY. NOTICE WHAT MAKES YOU HAPPY AND HOW YOU SPARKLE WHEN IN THE APPRECIATION OF IT.

5. PRAY AND ASK FOR DIRECTION IN BECOMING YOUR FULL POTENTIAL AS A COMMUNICATOR AND A LOVING PARTNER.

Chapter Ten

Playing the Perpetration Game!

Perpetrations are conclusions your mind believes are true and are not true. When the mind holds a judgment to be true, it supports the supposed validity by fabricating circumstances to prove it. When the truth is revealed, an immediate shift happens within the mind to support the real truth. A shift in belief immediately shifts your feelings about it.

Perpetrations are always easier to see in others than in yourself. A good example of a self-deception or perpetration is in the following story. Notice, in the example story, how the man's feelings completely shifted when the perpetration was exposed. Blame and anger shifted into compassion and forgiveness.

A Perpetration Uncovered

There was a man who had been wanting a new car for a long time. He saved and saved for his dream car. He finally got all the funds together to make a down payment. He was driving home on a busy freeway when all of a sudden a big rock came crashing down on the hood of his new car! You can imagine the outrage of the man. Here he was hurrying to where friends anxiously waited for him to show off his new car! All his life he had wanted this red Corvette convertible.

Angrily, he pulled off the road and ran after a young boy he saw running from the scene. He ran up a hill and down the other side with irate punishment going through his head. He couldn't wait to get his hands on the young vandal. Finally, he caught up with the boy, only to find him standing next to a younger boy laying on the ground holding his leg. "My brother broke his leg," he said. "I have been trying to get someone to stop for a long time by waving my hands and nobody would stop. So, I threw a rock to get your attention. I'm sorry for denting your car."

Immediately the anger changed to compassion. He now knew the truth. The truth set him free of the perpetration causing anger and allowed him to help the young boy. Picking up the small child, he went to the hospital.

The mind judges from the outward appearance.

Perpetrations happen from not having all of the information. As soon as the man saw the truth, he stopped reacting. Compassion is the natural state of truth, as is peace, love and understanding. In truth there is peaceful understanding.

**Is it possible that whenever we are feeling less
than a peaceful state, we are in a deception?**

For a two month period I traced every negative emotion that came up in me to a perpetration. My negative feelings disappeared with understanding their connection to difficult circumstances in my past.

A Woman's Perpetration with Her Mother

There was a perplexed woman who couldn't understand why her mother treated her father so badly. She grew up not liking her mother for this reason. She felt uncomfortable to be around her own mother, even as an adult. For ten years she had been trying to change her attitude toward her mother using many kinds of methods.

In a Kalos Process she was able to experience seeing through her mother's eyes and experienced her mother's feelings. She went back in the Process to the time when her mother was only five years old, to a time when her brothers molested her. The daughter found it difficult to believe that this could have happened to her mother, but stayed with the Process and found out even more information. Three brothers were involved. This behavior continued through her mother's teen years with one of the brothers. When her mother got married all of the "tapes" from those earlier years followed her. Insecurity, shame, anger and hostility attached to her sexuality. This became the BIG problem between Mom and Dad.

She took compassion on her mother through the information she gained, but questioned, "Could this really be true?" I told her that it really didn't matter. What really counted was how she felt toward her mother. Could she now understand why Mom treated Dad the way she did? The woman said she had gained so much insight and compassion for her mother that she could hardly wait to check out the story. Now she felt a connection that was never there before. The harsh judgments blocking her love was relieved.

127

Mom did love Dad. She had been caught up in a false belief. I call this false belief a PERPETRATION –SOMETHING WE THINK TO BE TRUE THAT ISN'T.

As soon as this woman walked into her home the phone rang. Guess who it was, Mom! Of course, the woman began asking questions. "Mom, were you ever molested when you were young?" Mom began to cry, "How did you ever find out? I have never told a soul, not even your father." Many times when you work on issues with a member of your family, they sense something is going on.

Not only does the Process affect the person personally involved, but also some other members of the family who have the same patterns.

The woman asked her mother about all the details that came up in the Kalos Process. Every detail was substantiated. The mother and daughter became closely connected from that time on. There was nothing to forgive. There was only the blessing of understanding. She now understood the cause of the tension and difficulties in her parents' marriage. Compassion for her mother's childhood took the place of resentment and grief. The perpetration was uncovered forever! The tension existing between them came from feelings carried over from a childhood trauma, not from lack of love. The truth set her free of separateness from her mother. The block to loving, understanding and communication was now gone. Incredible joy and gratitude were felt by both of them.

After a Kalos Process this is often what the participant feels and expresses. The word "Kalos" (meaning beautiful) was chosen because so often people would exclaim, "The Process is so beautiful." By removing misunderstanding, warm compassion allows forgiveness and love to flow. You can contrast this with many therapeutic processes, which leave the client feeling like they've gone through the mill.

An added benefit is that people are discovering:

Their problem is not because of the way someone is treating them, but because of their own early childhood programming.

Our reactionary mind assumes it knows what is going on now because of what went on in the past. This of course is absurd! The circumstances and people involved are entirely different now, only the feelings are the same. We cannot judge the present from the past. We can use the past to learn benefits for the future.

Perpetrations are Crimes within Our Own Mind

The commonly used dictionary definition of the word perpetration is committing a crime or an illegal act. My usage of the word is similar, but it is a crime in relation to ourself. It is an emotional crime against ourself or a self-deception. It was a crime that the two women in the story lived so many years estranged from one another, causing hurt, tension and countless difficulties. How sad it is that in many families there are similar situations of hurt and withheld love.

Perpetrations are Built on Fear

Perpetrations are deceptions we think are true that aren't or something we think we should do and don't. They form from misunderstandings and misjudgments. Fear is their foundation.

In the above example of a perpetration, the daughter had a devastating but unwarranted FEAR that her mother did not love her father. False fears come upon us out of the mind's compulsive need to avoid discomfort. The very thing she wanted to avoid happened only in her own mind. She thought that her mother did not love her dad. She then acted out a role and built evidence in her own mind of its validity and hated her mother for something that did not exist!

There is a survival mechanism within the mind that needs approval and desperately needs to be right. Before having all the needed information, the mind in haste may draw conclusions prematurely. Then everything becomes evidence to back up this conclusion and prove itself right. The secret, original decision, becomes buried under justifiable evidence (i.e. Mom doesn't love Dad).

There are Secrets within Perpetrations

I was three years old when I ran out into the street, almost getting hit by a car. Out of love, coupled with fear, my father grabbed me and gave me a spanking. He never wanted me to run in the street ever again! He acted angrily toward me, instead of holding me and telling me how afraid he was and how much he loved me.

In my heart, the subconscious mind, I made a decision about the incident with great emotion. "Dad doesn't really love me or he wouldn't scream at me and spank me. I didn't do anything wrong!" The secret decision, "Dad doesn't love me," began to rule my relationship with my Dad. This hidden decision was compounded with any new situations, where I proved I was right.

The mind begins to interpret everything as evidence to support the "truth" of the decision.

"Dad doesn't love me, so he lets my sister sit by him in the car. He takes my brothers camping and not me. He doesn't hear me when I talk to him." The list goes on and on with justification upon justification until Dad doesn't have a chance. With all this evidence to prove I am right, the relationship deteriorates and I feel worse and worse around my Dad.

With hidden emotions my mind created proof that it was right. It became an antenna, on guard around Dad, to interpret all of his actions. This way my mind felt safe in a world where it believed Dad loved the others much more than me.

The mind must be right to survive. So the more evidence it can gather to be right is all the better.

Proof after proof built in my survival-driven mind, all based upon a lie. I deceived myself into thinking that Dad didn't love me. This was a false assumption, a perpetration!

He yelled and spanked me because of his deep concern for my safety. He loved me so much it frightened him. He wanted to make sure I learned a lesson and never endangered myself like that again. He was shaken and reacted quickly without stopping to explain his feelings.

I judged the outward behavior, which felt cruel and inappropriate to me. I decided it was not safe to be close to him for he was mean to me when I needed him, and I was frightened too. I misunderstood at a deep level and a perpetration was born. In a Kalos Process, I got to look at the situation through my father's eyes. I got to see what he saw, feel what he felt and understand what was really going on. Dad really did love me!

Our minds would prefer being right than happy.

Once a decision is made in the inner mind with intense emotion attached, it becomes the rule of action from that time forth. My inner decision made me feel on guard around Dad. In this way my mind felt safe in a world where it believed Dad loved the others more than he loved me.

Our mind works diligently to keep us comfortable, and becomes very uncomfortable to find out it is wrong! Therefore, our minds go to great length to keep us right. The mind would rather be right than happy because being right is comfortable and being wrong is not. The mind would rather fight for its rights than submit to someone else being right. To take real joy in the happiness of others being right and us being wrong is beyond the mind.

The Mind is Designed for Self-Preservation

You did survive your childhood, otherwise you wouldn't be reading this book. Our minds serve us well, for what they are designed to do. With more understanding they can serve us even better. **Our minds can support reprogramming.** As soon as the mind discovers an error, it quickly makes changes to support being right in a new way.

The mind quickly responds to new and better truth and then acts to prove it. As we use our minds to explore new truths, we can re-define self-preservation and *ultimately what comfort really is.* A temporary discomfort is worth the long-term comfort of personal accomplishment and spiritual attainment.

You Can Heal the Past!

You can re-educate your mind on past dysfunctional beliefs by going back and re-experiencing them, uncovering the perpetration and releasing buried emotions and pain.

You will be able to see a benefit for every programmed deception and appreciate your learning experience. For instance, my feeling unloved was the driving force for me to understand how to love unconditionally. A benefit appears just like a rainbow at the end of every storm. Adversity can build strength.

In this way, your mind can serve you well. Not as the master but as servant, giving you "wake-up" calls when danger is present. Through the Spirit, you can renew your mind into the Mind of Christ. Whatever resentments you hold from the past colors your present experiences. Resentment is dark and burdensome. It is a major cause of emotional blocks, which will need to be cleared for good health. All negative emotions expose perpetrations.

The Kalos Process Heals Perpetrations and Releases Us from Dysfunctional Patterns

Through the Kalos Process, you can clear misinformation from your mind to see clearly. One of the best ways of doing this is going back to when the problem began. In the Process you determine what the perpetration is. You go into the other person's head and look through their eyes to see what was actually going on. You can feel the feelings they had at the time and experience the hidden love that was really there.

After you have been through a Kalos Process, you may wonder whether the information you experienced was really true. People have checked out the information and found it surprisingly accurate, such as the woman in the previous story. It is wonderful to see how new understanding can unblock emotions from the body. Misunderstandings are set straight in both the conscious and the subconscious mind. A long-standing pattern can be broken as healing takes place.

Patterns develop from perpetrations. Patterns of distrust, manipulation, loneliness, anxiety and failure can plague our lives. Through the Kalos Process, we can free ourselves from emotional pains.

Every Negative Emotion has a Perpetration Attached

I have experimented with perpetrations to see if every negative emotion, such as self-pity or anger, had a perpetration attached. What I found was:

Every time I had a feeling that was less than love and gratitude, it came from a perpetration.

I also discovered how often I deceived myself and others. I played out false roles and expectations, laboring to not disturb anyone. These perpetrations formed as a result of my running from my fear of not being loved.

Our First Demonstration of Love

When you experience being loved for the very first time (usually from mother and father), it makes an impression in your mind that follows you to adulthood. Watching your parents interact teaches you how to give and receive love. If your early experience of love is disconnected, uncaring, or "not there," it can affect all of your following relationships.

For example: Mary's father left her mother when Mary was only six months old. She never got to know him since he only showed up once in a while and then left again. Her first model of love was from a man who kept leaving her. As she grew up, every time she'd have a male companion he would leave. Each marriage would end in a divorce. She came to a workshop afraid of getting into another unsuccessful relationship.

In a Kalos Process Mary went back to her childhood to speak out the feelings she had locked in at the age of six months, before she had speech. What she discovered surprised her. Dad really did love her and was sorry to leave her behind. She saw how the erroneous perpetration had programmed her life. Ending her hatred toward her father, she resolved her distrust of men. She is now in a relationship that is mutually satisfying, expressive and committed.

Speaking Out Your Feelings is Part of the Release

Programming that occurs before speech, becomes locked in the body and hidden away. A satisfying relief is experienced when this is released. A light, open feeling of gratitude fills the empty space.

People who have difficulty in speaking their feelings usually had deep stress before the age of speech.

There are perpetrations that begin very early in life and become a pattern of behavior.

These behavioral patterns go unnoticed by the individual having them. Other people can see them quite easily. I call them "blind spots." They can cover or color one's actions so well that the real problem goes unnoticed.

As an example: Darla was always having problems with her children verbally abusing her. She tried talking to them and sharing her feelings, being very careful not to accuse them. After years of frustrating attempts, she decided to avoid all conversations with them. She decided to stop being "walked on" any more. This created a bigger separation from her family. She felt alone and misunderstood. She felt worthless to her family, instead of the closeness she so much desired.

This programming of being misunderstood and valueless went back to when she was very young. Her beliefs developed into a pattern of expectancy to be treated that way. Without realizing it she set others up to treat her in a certain way so that she could be right. This only strengthens the unwanted pattern with justifications, making the real deception harder to reach. When Darla saw her pattern she could then take responsibility for how her children treated her. "Know the truth and the truth shall set you free," still works. Her problem was not how her children spoke to her. It was how she handled the situation when they spoke. She had to stop supporting that expected behavior with her own reactive programming. Seeing how their language was how they manipulated their world, including her, she then CHOSE to respond in a loving, creative way. Their game had nothing to do with her. (Maybe it's no coincidence that her game played right into theirs.) She became a much better listener to understand her children's needs, the very act she wanted of them! If you really want to know your problem, look at what bothers you the most in your own family.

Darla's Perpetration Game

Her Pattern: Feeling misunderstood and of no value. (This was a result of her interpreting verbal abuse from childhood.)

Her Perpetration: She was unlovable, valueless. (Her way of expressing the false belief that there was something wrong with her.)

The Pay Off: Some attention and recognition, even though it was negative, like crumbs from the table of family love. She got to be right about being unlovable and valueless.

The Cost: Physical and emotional illness. Liver dysfunction relating to resistance to change. Sadness and loneliness from disconnection to family members.

Is It Worth It?: No, the cost is too great!

Her Compensation For Believing The Perpetration:

She over-involved herself in her children's lives to the point of giving huge amounts of time and substance. She looked for every possible way to be loved and needed.

The Benefit: She has become an extraordinary giver. She has learned many useful ways to care for and assist those in need. She has spent her life seeking new ways to support people in the healing process to be of more value! Great, but there is no satisfaction in the compensation.

Declaration Of TRUTH: "I am a valuable, loving person who listens and responds well to other people's needs."

This is a true statement. She is a valuable, caring person who listens well to the needs of others and responds appropriately, especially to her own children. Your declaration must be true.

Once the mind sees the perpetration it can respond in truth. This may require months of remembering to support and reprogram the mind to end the former pattern. When you realize you are paying too much (cost) for what you get back (your compensation), your mind supports you to "*tell the truth.*"

You can get stuck in the compensation, as well as the game. When you do, there may be difficulty in recognizing it. Keep remembering that even feelings of compulsion, the need to do good, etc. are driven by the mind and have a perpetration attached.

Sometimes it happens surprisingly fast; other times stubbornness needs releasing, and being replaced with a commitment to transform.

You can Speed up the Renewing Process

The process can be sped up by doing a Cross Crawl Exercise to reprogram the mind. It is amazing how your feelings can change by becoming honest about your intentions. A Cross Crawl Exercise can integrate your intention to a deeper level, to where it becomes a more natural way of being.

While seeing yourself as successful in whatever is your Declaration of Truth, do Cross Crawl exercises standing in place or on a trampoline. This looks like walking in place and swinging your arms the way you do when you walk. Then move your eyes in a large circle, like a huge clock, while humming. Rotate your eyes in both directions, clockwise and counterclockwise. *Think and speak the TRUTH and feel* the results come into being.

Do these exercises for 2 or 3 minutes daily for two weeks. You can use this exercise anytime you fall into negative emotions or compulsive behavior. Go through each step of the Perpetration Game and write it down. You really are in charge of your life. You can choose to support other people to treat you well instead of poorly. **You can win at the Perpetration Game!**

Experiencing Our Experience and Sharing it can Prevent New Perpetrations from Forming

You can prevent new perpetrations from forming by willingly experiencing the discomforts of the moment. Feel what's there, instead of judging it, suppressing it and running away from it. You can keep your ears and heart open. Then open your mouth and share what you're thinking and feeling. In other words, just acknowledge your discomfort without blaming others for creating it. **Own being the source of the feeling.**

Your life transforms as you stop choosing comfort over expressing truth. The mind's way of blaming surrenders to being a vehicle for Spirit to express through. You can then respond easily to the calling God puts in your heart, whether it is comfortable or not! Joy is the ability to be happy in any situation.

Highlights

* Perpetrations are hidden agendas (beliefs) based upon an untruth. Since the mind made the decision, it must prove it is right. The mind creates experiences to justify itself. For example, the agenda Mary had that if a man loved her, he would leave her. This can create unresolved emotions and constant upsets.

* During upsets, perpetrations are programmed into the mind and secretly rule your life.

* Justifications are encrusted upon one another to bolster the (false) decision. Your mind would rather be RIGHT than happy.

* Examine every feeling that is not peaceful, loving or contented and you will find a perpetration behind it. Something hidden is going on.

* Making something so important that it becomes a need causes deceptions to take place. Needs are important, while preferences don't have expectations attached. When we take a second look at past situations, we may wonder WHY we made it so important.

* The survival mechanism of the mind causes fear of not enough. The mind is programmed to NEED more, better, or different. When this is understood and watched you are then ready to go beyond the programming and allow WHO you are to make your decisions. The WHO you are (spirit)

understands your purpose and is not living only to be comfortable.

* When you renew your mind, the judging turns into understanding. Your needs turn into preferences. You can then go behind the behavior to the underlying intent and respond to that which is positive.

* Love is all there is. Perhaps, to believe there is any act outside of love is to experience a perpetration. We are not short of love, only short on the ability to express it in a mature way.

* You can speed up your healing by doing a Cross Crawl exercise while repeating and imaging your declaration of truth. This supports the reprogramming of the mind.

* Experiencing our experiences and sharing them can help to prevent perpetrations from forming anew.

Participant's Page

Play the Perpetration Game!
Locate Your Own Pattern!
Use Darla's Case As An Example.
Happy Discovering!

If you would like to play this game to discover a pattern in your own life, answer the following questions. (Writing them down will make it easier to examine):

1. WHAT IS YOUR BIGGEST COMPLAINT ABOUT YOUR LIFE? What is the pattern that keeps repeating itself and leaving you frustrated?

2. WHAT IS THE NEGATIVE DECISION YOU MADE ABOUT YOURSELF? This is the perpetration. (i.e. I am not . . ., I can't . . .)

3. WHAT IS YOUR PAY OFF? In what way do you get to be right about your inability to be who you want to be? What discomfort do you try to protect yourself from? (i.e. I avoid . . ., I get to . . .)

4. WHAT IS IT COSTING YOU? How is your life being affected by this? (i.e. My health . . ., happiness . . .)

5. IS IT WORTH IT? (Yes or no)

6. WHAT DO YOU DO TO COMPENSATE FOR YOUR PERPETRATION, FOR FAILING AT WHAT YOU

REALLY WANT TO BE? (Because of not . . . , I must do
. . . to compensate.)

7. HOW HAS THIS BENEFITTED YOUR LIFE? What
special gifts and talents have you developed for believing
this lie? What are you known for being exceptional at? Be
honest, not shy. You have certainly achieved some skills
because of needing to compensate for feeling like a failure
in the other area. (Notice how Darla developed some useful
skills in helping others.)

8. NOW MAKE A STATEMENT OF THE TRUTH
(Declaration of Truth)! YOU DO NOT HAVE TO COM-
PENSATE ANYMORE. YOU CAN *CHOOSE* TO SEE
AND ACT UPON THE "TRUTH" OF THE MATTER.
(i.e. I am . . .)

Practice your special statement while doing the Cross
Crawl Exercise and watch how much faster you integrate it
into your normal behavior. You can transform your life no
faster than you can get honest. Don't expect your pattern to
change over-night. It requires practice. Trying to stop your
pattern only makes it worse. Accept it, appreciate what it
has done for you, own it - choose it for now.

Chapter Eleven

Spiritual Awakening Needed in Our World Today!

Being in a Mature Relationship with God

What is the difference between being a relative and being in a close relationship? It is comparable to the difference between a close friend and an acquaintance. What a difference there is in these two very similar words – relative and relationship. Is God a distant relative or your closest friend?

Most relatives are only seen now and then or not at all our whole lifetime. They are people we hear about (particularly if they have done something noteworthy, whether good or bad). There are close relatives with whom we develop relationships and there are distant relatives rarely seen. Are you simply related to or in relationship with God?

Relationships involve, evolve and are a continuum of closeness and caring.

Closeness means you are understood and accepted. It's being in the space of someone else's love and true intent. It's understanding their heart and life purpose. It's even making that purpose your own when you are together.

Spirit Gives Life Meaning

Spiritual values give human life its essential meaning and dignity. There is a great need for spiritual awakening in our world today. In the Higher Consciousness of Spirit, we find lasting peace and happiness. Every being is sustained by Spirit. All people are of this one dynamic family.

What is SPIRIT? Spirit comes from the word "espirit" or in Latin "spiritus" meaning breath, air, life, soul. "God breathed into the nostrils of Adam and he became a living Being." (Whether taken literally or allegorically, God gives Life.)

One of the mysteries of the ages is to understand ourselves and our relationship to God. The dictionary calls spirit – "The vital principle in man animating our body and the mediator between our body and mind." Spirit is also called essence and our pervading temperament or tone. Whatever you call spirit, it is our ALIVENESS. It is WHO we are!

We have a body, but are not that body. We have a mind, but are not that mind. We are spirit, created in the image of God with all the attributes of God. Our body is a temple for the living God to dwell in. You can destroy your body, but your spirit is forever!

Everyone experiences God's Spirit in their own way. Some have structured rituals and others live in constant awareness of "The Presence." We all can relate personally and individually to God and receive the needed guidance and wisdom for our lives.

Letters to God

The question I hold in my heart is: "God, what is YOUR purpose for my life? What am I here for?" You might, this moment, write out some questions for God, and then let God answer you. I learned this technique from my close friend, Terry, who shared his letters to God with me. I have appreciatively corresponded this way with God ever since. There are many questions that are clarified and I feel a glorious peace each time I finish. It doesn't take the place of prayer and meditation, it only enhances it.

Just write on a piece of paper: Dear God. Then write your heart out. Ask any question you want. Pour out your feelings and express your doubts. Tell it all. When finished, write: Dear (your name). Then receive God's answer through your own hand. This process has meant much to me, especially when I've been overwhelmed with too much going on. It is a breath of fresh air as it clears my mind of unwanted stress, giving me insight and understanding, correction and love. The peace that follows, when I receive my answer back, is food for my soul.

Everyone has Their Own Way to Listen to God

You can tell how deeply you love people by the amount of time you want to spend with them. I find God's Presence always here. Anytime I look inside, God is there. Anytime I need help or advice, God is there. *I have learned to trust inner guidance knowing "All things work for my good."*

147

There was a time when I was tormented from not knowing how to listen to God.

When I was thirteen years old and living in a foster home, God gave me a clear audible voice to answer my requests. I needed that in my insecure world. Other times it's a voice in my mind that answers me, then shortly someone will say the same thing. Later I may read an article which confirms this as an additional witness. It will help you develop a deeper relationship with God and enable you to have clear communication that builds confidence. Wouldn't it be awful to love someone and not be able to communicate with them?

"What is Your Will for Me in this Situation?"

IS IT GOD OR MY MIND?

Once I couldn't figure out if I was hearing God direct me or my mind directing me. So I decided to ask God to make it easier for me to tell which was which. My mind would get confused with so many conflicting thoughts. My heartfelt sense was usually clearer.

I realized God could take my heart and put His Will into it, so then I could just follow my heart!

It was difficult for a time to accept that God wanted me to have the desires of my heart. Now I give thanks for the joy and clarity this has brought into my life. And, contrary to the God of my youth, I discovered a God that loved to say yes!

Personal revelation is an individual matter. God is no "respecter of persons" the Bible says, and I believe it is true. God speaks to all people in their own language and culture. I really appreciate that I can trust God to guide and direct all people everywhere. My prayer is that everyone listen.

God cares about everyone, no matter who they are!

The more I trust God, the more I see God working in the world. I notice that just about everyone I know relates to God in a little different way, but through the same kind of love. Sometimes it appears that everyone is worshiping a different God because they believe in different doctrines. There are so many beliefs, yet God is big enough for all. Everyone can have a personal relationship with God and experience **Unconditional Love.**

God's Love is Different

I like the way the Greeks defined four kinds of love, using four different words. We in the United States have only one word - LOVE. It is wonderful how the ancient Greeks knew God's Love was different. His Love is unconditional, beyond needing to be returned. It is a love that could even embrace an enemy. They called His Love– *Agape*.

"Agape" is not conditional upon being loved back. It is not limited by mental programming, but it is of the unlimited Spirit. In contrast, everything the mind does is conditional to keep us safe, right and to preserve our lives. "Agape" is spiritual love, patient, not easily provoked and free to express without conditions attached. To express what it is not, is easier than to express what agape is.

I remember when I was verbally attacked by a person who felt I was a threat to her. The deep love I felt while accusations were hurled against me was astonishing. I actually felt compassion for her upset. What I was experiencing was agape love.

The Three Conditional Loves

We call the following types of loves conditional because they dissipate when not returned.

1. Philia – Friendships, Brotherly love
2. Pia – Family love
3. Eros – Erotic love

Have you ever wondered how you can be so in love only to "fall" out of it again? Have you wondered how families can be enemies to each other, or how friends cease to be friends? It is because all of these kinds of love are conditional upon receiving love back. We call it the "You scratch my back and I'll scratch yours" routine.

When the mind's loving gets uncomfortable, it begins to dissipate and can even turn into hatred. This can never happen to spiritual love. Spiritual love never fails. It bears all things and endures all things. It is the very love, called charity that Paul spoke of in I Corinthians 13.

"Love never fails." Though: prophecy shall fail, tongues shall cease, knowledge shall vanish away.

Paul makes it clear that it doesn't matter what great virtues we have or even what great gifts we have, even the faith to move mountains. If we do not love (agape), we are nothing!

I believe nothing can be clearer than this. **Without love we really are nothing.** I cannot conceive living without love. My heart goes out to those who live in remote loneliness, not knowing how to express their love.

Maybe we don't have a shortage of love. It is that we do not express that love in a mature way. How many people have you hugged today? How many have you said, "I love you" to today? When we are all willing to express love openly, we will see much transformation on the planet.

When teachers too, can reach out and hug their students, and treat them like children of God who want and need love, then maybe we will have crossed a big bridge to living A SPIRITUAL LIFE.

We are All Beings of Love – Created in God's Image

If this be true, why is it so difficult to express it? Why do people fall into such immature behavior? Why is love professed one moment only to dissipate the next? What causes all this? Don't worry, it's only your mind momentarily feeling insecure. Remember, you are not your mind! It is only programming. You are spirit!

You can live and love in the Spirit as fast as the speed of thought! It's your choice, for you are love!

Highlights

* Spiritual awakening is needed and possible in our world today by being in a mature relationship with God.

* Spiritual values give life essential meaning and dignity.

* Our spirit is the vital principle animating our bodies and the mediator between our bodies and minds.

* Every one can relate to God personally and individually, no matter what set of beliefs they may have.

* You can write a letter to God and let Him answer you. Letters open the line of communication and create the space for love and peace.

* Listen to God speak to you. Everyone has their own way to listen. Trust your inner guidance. You will be able to develop your own unique way to interact with God.

* Giving your heart to God makes it easier to be guided clearly.

* The Greeks describe four kinds of love: Philia, Pia, Eros and Agape. Agape is God's unconditional love.

* God's perfect love (Agape) loves unconditionally without strings attached.

* We are all BEINGS of love, created in God's image. We all have the potential to love maturely by choice.

* You can live and love in the Spirit at the speed of thought. It's your choice, because you are love.

Participant's Page

1. PLAN A TIME TO FEED AND DEVELOP YOUR SPIRITUAL POTENTIAL. This works best on a daily basis, such as before sleep or early in the morning. Short prayers throughout the day and/or a short meditation can sustain you spiritually in the midst of a demanding day. What can you commit to?

2. WRITE DOWN THE AREAS OF YOUR SPIRITUAL WALK YOU WANT TO FOCUS ON. Example: Prayer, meditation, inspirational reading, uplifting music, visits to shut-ins, teaching inspirational lessons. Be honest and don't commit to more than you can do. You can always increase with time.

3. FIND A "SPIRITUAL PARTNER" TO DISCUSS SPIRITUAL MATTERS WITH. MEET WITH OTHERS OF LIKE MIND AND SPIRIT. SUPPORT EACH OTHER IN YOUR SPIRITUAL WALK.

4. SEVERAL TIMES A DAY, STOP, LISTEN TO THE DIRECTION OF THE SPIRIT. YOU CAN ALWAYS ASK YOURSELF, "HOW WOULD GOD WANT ME TO RESPOND?"

5. LIVE IN THE PRESENT MOMENT (NOW) AS OFTEN AS YOU CAN. AS SOON AS YOU DISCOVER YOU AREN'T, YOU ARE!

6. WRITE DOWN A MOTTO ON A CARD OR PAPER SUCH AS, "BE KIND." PLACE IT WHERE IT RE- MINDS YOU DAILY OF A SPIRITUAL QUALITY YOU WANT TO EXPAND IN YOUR LIFE.

These suggestions are not to add to your burdens, but to lessen them. They are to support you in being the spiritual giant you are intended to be. By all means, be playful with it. Jesus said, "My burden is light, my yoke is easy." Your intentions for your spiritual walk will do much to support your journey. Make some goals to expand your relationship with God.

C h a p t e r   T w e l v e

Lighten Up and Be Happy!

Some people get so heavy about enlightenment. Life is too important to take it seriously! Enlightenment is simply having a renewed, illumined mind. Life becomes lighter and easier when you aren't bogged down in the burdens of right living, right knowing and right thinking. It's just your mind that needs to be right. Why not lighten up!

How?

A way of doing this is by *not taking ourselves too seriously.* If we make allowances for our own silly "off the mark" behavior, we will do the same for others. We usually judge ourselves more harshly than others, so lighten up with yourself! Get honest about what you are about! Your mind can keep you burdened with worry about whether you are doing "it" right!

Just notice what you do, when you do it.

What you think, when you have those thoughts.

And how you feel, when you feel that way.

Lighten Up by Raising Your Thoughts

You can up-level any thought or feeling at any time by appreciating what is going on in the moment. Pretend you are choosing what is happening. Then look for the benefit involved. Being aware of how you function in relation to life can be FUN! It can increase discovery and potentialize your experience!

Express More Love!

Another way of lightening up about your life and increasing your joy is to express more love. We all have at our disposal the ability to share love in a mature way. We can share and care in fun and meaningful ways! Start with BEING WITH, WHO YOU ARE WITH, WHEN YOU ARE WITH THEM. Repeat the last sentence slowly to get it.

When I am with who I am with, time stands still. Life becomes a new experience, not the same old boring repetitions in new content. Try looking at people right into their eyes, the windows to their soul. Practice just being there and listening to them. Hear their heart. Listen to their need. Be there! Notice how you feel. Come alive and share, then listen. You have two ears and only one mouth. Maybe this means we are to listen twice as much as we speak.

Express Love through Touch; A Gentle Touch or Heart-Felt Hug Can save the Day!

We can touch each other through thoughts and beliefs and feelings, but not until we touch physically does it really affect our health. Research was done by Dr. David Bresler,

156

Director of the Pain Control Unit at UCLA, which led to his recommending bear-hugging.

"I often tell my patients to use hugging as a part of their treatment for pain. Being held is enormously therapeutic," he says.

Hugging is a miracle medicine that can relieve many physical and emotional problems, the experts are saying. Researchers have also discovered that hugging can help you live longer, protect you against illness, relieve depression and stress, strengthen family relationships and even help you sleep without pills.

Dr. Robert Rynearson, Psychiatry Department Chairman, White Clinic, Temple, Texas, said, "I'm convinced that the tender embrace can prevent or cure a host of different problems. A hug can have an astonishing therapeutic effect by providing a sense of companionship and happiness."

"Researchers discovered that when a person is touched, the amount of hemoglobin in their blood increases significantly," said Helen Colton, author of "The Joy of Touching." Hemoglobin is a part of the blood that carries vital supplies of oxygen to all organs of the body, including the heart and brain. An increase in hemoglobin tones up the whole body, helps prevent disease and speeds recovery from illness. A trained nurse, Pamela McCoy, R.N., Grant Hospital, Columbus, Ohio, said, "We found that people who are hugged or touched can often stop taking medication in order to get to sleep."

Speak Words of Love that Kindle Closeness

Your voice is a valuable way to express love. Even though words may come slowly, you can express a kind thought. If you will place yourself in someone else's shoes, you can relate to how they would want to hear it. Expressing love in the form of appreciation allows words to flow easier. Sometimes words can get stuck in the throat because of fear they will not be received. Just notice your resistances then choose to express how you feel. Subtle layers of resistance may come up to be released, as we expand into our full potential of loving.

Some have a gift with words. It doesn't matter whether you have a gift or not. Everyone wants to hear words of love, no matter how you say them. It's saying them that counts. Who cares if they stutter out or squeak out in embarrassment. Who cares how lengthily or profoundly they are spoken. JUST SPEAK WORDS OF LOVE, HOWEVER, WHENEVER YOU CAN!

If there is a shortage of anything on this planet, it is the expressing of love in a mature way. It is time for our planet to "wake-up" and create the peace we all want. We can start today to EXPRESS LOVE FULLY; not as a burden, but to lighten up our lives!

Let's make the journey so much fun that it really doesn't matter when the journey is over. Who knows, maybe at the end of this one another awaits? And the next journey will add upon the ability we have right now to give and receive love.

In my challenge to you all to LIGHTEN UP, I present this story about the Host. It is one of my favorite stories that helps me to stay light about Enlightenment.

God the Host

Once upon a time there was a wonderful party! A beautiful place was created by the Host and thousands of special guests were invited there. All were invited to have a marvelous time, enjoying the games and other guests, as well as visiting with the Host.

No one needed to bring anything with them, because everything was provided by the Host. They just "showed up!" It was a wonderful party called Planet Earth.

Everything was Provided at the Party!

Every kind of food you can think of was available at the party and served with delight. Beautiful dishes and silverware were available as well as beautiful furnishings. The guests could use anything at the party they wanted. They could carry goodies around with them; or set up their own private collection, however they wanted. Clothes of all kinds were provided in all sizes, as well as toys and playthings to keep everyone amused.

No one, of course, would think of taking any of it with them when they left, as all belonged to the Host. Everyone came to the party with the intention and anticipation of having the time of their Life, a great time, a joyful celebration!

Not only was there an abundance of joy, but an abundance of everything at the party. Games of all kinds made the party fun and exciting. There were sports games, doctor games, nursing games, secretarial games, carpenter games, religious games, family games, money games, political games and even war games. Every type of game you could possibly think of was at the party. And the guests could even start a new game, if they preferred. All could express their creativity freely at the party.

"People are invited to have abundant joy," said the Host.

Some Got Too Serious at the Party!

Sometimes people got so involved in the game they would forget they were at a party. They would spend hours on end without stopping, overly anxious about the outcome. They even worried about what other guests thought about how they played the game. They'd get so intense, they'd faint!

"Life at the party is too valuable to take it seriously," the Host replied.

Still people got frustrated and worked up in a frenzy over little things in the games. Resentment, anger, frustration and guilt blocked the natural flow of Life energy in their bodies and caused them to get sick. Again and again the people forgot it was a big party to have a great time! They forgot they were a guest of the Host and didn't have to worry about anything.

Some Wanted to Serve at the Party

Some noticed other guests fainting and going unconscious at the party and asked the Host if they could help. They had become somewhat tired of the games and wanted to be of assistance. They wanted to do anything they could to make it a happy, memorable party for everyone. It didn't matter what the job was, as long as they served the Host. Happily, the Host agreed. It was a very big party and many could help. The Host assigned the jobs and gave them what they needed to accomplish them. How happy they felt to have an assignment from the Host!

All are Grateful to the Host for Providing the Party

Everyone who assisted at the party knew it was their own CHOICE and REQUEST to serve. Therefore, they did not need recognition. They were doing what THEY WANTED for the Host. Happily, they went about their work, gratefully doing what they wanted to SERVE THE HOST. When someone went unconscious, the servant got to **wake them up!** "What a privilege," they said, "I'm doing what I love to do." So they never needed thanks for assisting, instead, they thanked the Host.

When a guest received help, he thanked the Host for providing assistance at the party. He didn't think of thanking the servant, for the servant did it for the Host. All were being taken care of and ALL WERE GRATEFUL TO THE HOST.

"Whosoever helps with even the least of my guests, has actually done it unto me," said the Host.

A Spirit of Celebration Comes to the Party!

As more and more people became conscious of the games and stopped taking the party so seriously, a spirit of celebration came into the party that had not been there before. Feelings of joy and satisfaction permeated the games and filled the air with fun! They let go of making the game so important and realized their lives were too valuable for that. They took charge of their lives, surrendering to the purpose of the celebration and laughed much more!

Guest after guest celebrated with the Host and treated the other guests as the special people they were. Appreciation entered a new high as each realized just how MUCH the Host had provided. Divine Gratitude replaced the previous worry over the games, so much so that harmony flowed through their bodies. A calming balance came into their nervous systems and sickness was heard of no more.

As all recognized that they were loved and cared for at the party of the Host, a glorious shout went up to Heaven.

What a wonderful party!

Let's all give a toast!

Lighten up and Enjoy

The party of the Host!

The Host responded, *"A New Earth, like Heaven!"*

Highlights

* It is easy to get too heavy about Enlightenment. Don't get bogged down in doing everything right. Lighten up!

* We can lighten up by expressing more love. Be with who you are with, when you're with them.

* Express love through touch. Hugging is a miracle medicine that relieves many physical and emotional problems.

* Speak words of love. Take control of your tongue and express appreciation. Treat others in the way you want to be treated.

* Reminisce about the story of "The Host" to aid you to lighten up about enlightenment. Don't faint from making the games in life too important. Whatever you do or however you serve, do it for the Host.

Participant's Page

1. CHOOSE TO ENJOY YOUR LIFE. THE GREATEST GIFT YOU CAN GIVE YOUR FRIENDS AND FAMILY IS A HAPPY, LOVING ATTITUDE!

2. SET UP A PROGRAM TO SUPPORT YOUR SPIRITU-AL GROWTH.

3. MEET WITH OTHERS OF LIKE MIND TO CELE-BRATE AND SERVE THE HOST IN A MEANINGFUL WAY.

C o n c l u s i o n

Be Healed! And Stay Well!

TO BE HEALED IS A PROMISE BY GOD AND A
CHOICE BY EACH OF US.

STAYING WELL IS AN ONGOING EVENT OF
ALIGNING TO NATURAL LAWS, RENEWING THE
MIND AND LIVING A TRANSFORMED LIFE.

The ways to stay well are many. They will include
caring for yourself in THE FOUR BASIC areas of attitude,
nutrition, exercise, and environment. All have a bearing on
your health, with your attitude having the most effect.

**I find the only time a problem comes up is when I'm
upset. To resolve the problem, I immediately trace it and
clear it.**

DAILY, I take care of the basics: nutrition, exercise and
environment. This makes it easy to identify what attitude is
throwing my body out of balance. Quickly, I can then trace
the upset and clear it out.

When I see myself resisting one of these four areas, I just trace the resistance to its cause. Then I attend to it immediately.

The area of strength that supports me the most is my relationship to God.

To know that I am loved and looked after by a caring Being, gives me peace. It fills my heart with the great *attitude of gratitude*. Appreciating my life, my mate, my children, my career, etc. brings me high energy and health. Our attitude has a great deal to do with how we feel about life, ourselves and God. Notice how fast the body breaks down when you are not happy.

Expressing your unique Purpose adds MEANING to your life.

Until you are in touch with your Divine Purpose, life may lack the enthusiasm and zeal necessary for well-being. Your Purpose for living has already prepared you for a mission in life. Realizing it and living it brings joy. You have special gifts and talents that make you unique and valuable. You can elevate your energy and vitality by accomplishing your Purpose. Knowing that your life is making a difference in someone else's life is motivating and uplifting! Remember how much energy you got when a friend called and invited you to do your favorite activity? Energy fills a tired body when you are doing what you love to do. If you are too tired to do the things you love, you need some emotional clearing and physical healing immediately!

I describe purpose as being an "ongoing event that always has to do with others." How you manifest this purpose is your mission, for you and God to decide.

Expressing your Full Potential is living your Purpose moment to moment. You choose your thoughts, whether conditional or unconditional. You choose how you spend your time.

In the World, but Not of the World

We live in the world, but are not of the world. The world is made up of physical laws that sometimes seem in opposition to the spiritual world. Yet when we take those laws to their source, we meet the inherent harmony in the universe. Laws of physics express universal harmonics. Science and religion are not in opposition to each other. God created natural laws and expresses harmony and balance through all creation.

Manifesting who (spirit) and what (love) we are in the finite universe (matter) is our underlying challenge. Maybe we are a bit clumsy in the way we express the WHO we are. Maybe this is the area that needs the most understanding and developing. We can live in the experience of our FULL POTENTIAL as the Holy Spirit is the director of our Life.

We are not our bodies or our minds. We are far beyond this. We are spirit, created in the image of God. We have the attributes of God, also called "fruits." Fruit is something that comes only from mature trees. Young trees do not bear fruit. Love, joy, peace, patience, kindness, goodness, faithfulness, gentleness and self-control are God-given capacities to express our full potential.

By surrendering our will to the Will of God, we allow Spirit to express itself in our lives. This is what maturity really is. Through God's Spirit, or the Holy Spirit, we can express maturely. This keeps us well! This keeps us in joy and interested in life. God's Spirit is the very "Tree of Life" referred to in the Garden of Eden. We can BE HEALED and STAY WELL!

As a HEALTHY person we can go forth in a greater way to live the Purpose meant for our lives; the very Purpose we came to live at this particular time.

What is God Calling You to do with Your Life?

"What you are is God's gift to you.
What you become is your gift to God."

I get really excited to see people healed. I love to see people set free of bondage of all types. I am especially excited to see people happy, really happy and feeling empowered from on high. My heart delights in seeing people with a confidence in God, as they manifest their Purpose.

I get excited when I see people fulfilling their dreams. I love to see families loving each other. Inner healing is the most exciting to me, because that has been the most painful part of my life. I have had some severe, painful, injuries; but most pain does not last. Although pain of the heart can go on for years, interfering with happiness and joy, without joy there is no PURPOSE at all.

Once you live in harmony with God and in the confidence it brings, you never want to live any other way. Commitment to serving God opens doors to dynamically fulfilling your potential.

Being Part of a Bigger Picture: Co-creating

I seek to be a part of a BIGGER picture that takes this healing work to the world, to all people of all cultures. There are so many places in the world where we could turn the health of an area around very rapidly by training groups of Health Facilitators. Much of what I am doing now is to train others to do this work professionally. I love being involved in a movement to improve the quality of life for all.

You can Be Healed!
You can assist others to Be Healed!
You can choose to live your Full Potential!

I LOVE YOU, BE HEALED!

Epilogue

The Next Step

You will want to investigate the Healing Manuals referred to in this book. They include a step by step technology to enable you to uncover and resolve your problems.

In Book Two, the Kalos Process is explained in detail along with the principles behind each step. Examples of healings are recorded to support your own process. You can enjoy experimenting on yourself or add to the class material after taking a Kalos Seminar. We are committed to supporting your healing process in every way we can.

In Book Three you will learn how to do Muscle Response Testing (MRT). You will need some hands-on practice to be able to use all of this Manual. It is designed to start a beginner and to move the more advanced student to new levels of results. This book really gets down to tracing a problem to its cause with several modalities to align your body and place it into a "healing mode." A healing mode happens when all the systems of the body are renewing and repairing themselves at the fastest rate possible.

By going through the techniques and doing the muscle testing, you are able to actually fine-tune what is optimum health for your body. You can test foods and supplements, a dietary cleanse, structural alignment, etc.

Attending Kalos Seminars will support you in pursuing your health-related and purposeful goals. You will have the opportunity to do hands-on practicing with professional guidance. You can send for free information using the order form at the back of this book.

The focus is on teaching you the tools of how you can take care of your own body. If you have projects, learn the material and go for results. You can use the methods at home on yourself or with your family. You can also incorporate them into clinical practice. Many health professionals are now using these or similar methods.

The object is to support the body's vital energy and immune system to be as efficient as possible by resolving the cause and getting rid of the blocks that get in the way of recovery. You can heal. You can be happy. You can live a fruitful life.

God is Blessing You Now!

ABOUT THE AUTHOR

Valerie Seeman Moreton is a graduate of the International College of Naturopathy and has been practicing wholistic healing, lecturing, and training students for over twenty years. She has intensively researched to find ways the body could heal itself through proper physical, mental and spiritual balance. In 1969, she began practicing as a nutritional consultant, while continuing her studies in pathology and bio-mechanics of the human body. Interning through her husband's medical/surgical practice gave her the opportunity to explore natural healing methods under orthodox supervision. As a result, the clinic's need for surgeries among its patients was greatly reduced and Valerie was proclaimed a "natural healer."

She expanded her studies of nutrition and herbology through Dr. Henry G. Bieler, M.D. and Dr. Bernard Jensen, N.D., D.C. By working with patients that the medical profession could no longer help, she was able to find additional ways to assist the body to heal itself. Next, she added the technology of "Creative Healing Massage" to alleviate pain and inflammation, then received her M.T. degree from Alpha Massage School, San Mateo, California in 1973.

Her studies with Stan Malstrom, N.D. and Dr. John Christopher motivated her to start lecturing on health, nutrition, herbology and Applied Kinesiology. In 1976, she became certified to teach the "Touch for Health" (TFH) Workshops. She taught hundreds of students TFH and advanced healing techniques on how to relieve pain, overcome allergies and release stress. She received special coaching from some of the most gifted people in Kinesiology, including; George Goodheart, D.C., John Thie, D.C.,

Sheldon Deal, D.C., Gordon Stokes, Daniel Whitesides, and Paul Dennison.

In 1978, Valerie founded Wholistic Health Education in El Dorado County, California. Through research with students and patients she developed many new methods for using Muscle Response Testing (MRT) to communicate with the body at much deeper levels and trace any problem to its source. In her continuing aim to integrate the body, mind and spirit in the healing process she became certified in One Brain, 1983; and Advanced One Brain, 1984, to work effectively with dyslexia and learning disabilities.

Valerie assisted in the development of the RFA (Relaxed Focused Attention) Process, a simplified method of helping to reprogram the subconscious mind to a perpetual positive attitude. The Process focused on clearing unwanted emotional blocks from early childhood by "seeing the truth" to be set free. The Kalos Process evolved out of the RFA Process, adding the "maturing of the mind" part.

With teaching as her major goal and joy, in 1986 she founded what is now Kalos Seminars International. With a commitment to healing and transformation, she has taught thousands of lay people and professionals how the body/mind works, how to relieve pain, how to overcome disease and how to take charge of their lives.

Index

175

KALOS™ PUBLISHING

Envisioning a Transformed World

QUICK ORDER FORM - A New Day in Healing
1-800-77-KALOS

With Credit Card: **Phone:** (800) 775-2567 **Fax:** (619) 748-7081
Postal: Payment must be included with order
P. O. Box 270817-1, San Diego, CA, 92128-2817, USA

Please Print   Phone _____

Name _____

Address _____

City _____ State _____ Zip _____

MAIL ORDER DISCOUNTS	CA RES. SALES TAX	SHIPPING/HANDLING
One Book, $12.00 (U.S.A.)	$0.78	$2.00
2-10 Books, $10.00 each	$0.65 each	$1.00 each

❑ *Please forward a copy of A NEW DAY IN HEALING with a gift card saying (Please Print)*

A Gift from: _____

To: _____

Address _____

City _____ State _____ Zip _____

Payment: ❑ Check   ❑ Visa   ❑ Master Card
Card Number _____
Name on Card _____
Expiration Date _____/_____/_____   _____
                                                       Signature

Please send me_____book(s) @ $_____ = $ _____
CA only sales tax _____book(s) $_____ = $ _____
Shipping/Handling   Total = $ _____

I understand that I may return book(s) in saleable condition within 30 days for a full refund for any reason, no questions asked.

❑   Please keep me informed about Kalos books, videos/cassettes, seminars, and training.